Managing Diabetes on a Budget

$

A project of the
American Diabetes Association

$

By Leslie Y. Dawson

Sandy Weinrauch, *Senior Editor*

Publisher
Susan H. Lau

Editorial Director   Editor
Peter Banks   Sherrye Landrum

AMERICAN DIABETES ASSOCIATION
1660 Duke Street
Alexandria, VA 22314

Library of Congress Cataloging-in-Publication Data
Dawson, Leslie Y. (Leslie Young)
Managing diabetes on a budget/by Leslie Y. Dawson.
p. cm
"A project of the American Diabetes Association."
Includes index.
ISBN 0-945448-53-8
1. Diabetes—Economic aspects. I. American Diabetes Association.
II. Title.
RC660.D38   1995
362.1'96462—dc20   95-16705
                                          CIP

Managing Diabetes on A Budget

$

TABLE OF CONTENTS

Acknowledgments

$

I have had diabetes and periodic bouts of low income for many years. I have gleaned money-saving ideas from professionals working in health care, pharmaceuticals, insurance, medical supply, and government. Everyone I talked to saw a need for this book and gladly contributed to it. I thank them and the many people with diabetes who have shared their budget-saving ideas with me over the years.

Don and Nancy Dawson's on-going battle with diabetes has inspired my faith that one can lead an active and happy life *with* the disease.

Special thanks go to Senior Editor Sandy Weinrauch, MSW, for her experience, guidance, and advice with this book. She helped it take form and direction.

I would also like to thank the following people for reading and reviewing the book and for offering more good suggestions to be included in the text: Phyllis Barrier, MS, RD, CDE; Peggy M. Batchelor; Eleanor Lorden, RN, MS, CNS, CDE; Lois Lipsett, PhD; Dolly Daniel, RN, CDE; Barbara J. Maschak-Carey, RNCS, MSN, CDE; David B. Kelley, MD; Lisa Wheaton, MD; Renee Wall, MS, RD, CDE; Kathy Ford, ACSW, CSW; and Ann Stowell, RN, BSN, CETN.

Sherrye Landrum edited this manuscript and provided constant support, Orit Lowy Chicherio, Marjorie Weber, and Karen Ingle copyedited it. Stacey Wages designed and desktopped the pages. Heidi Fixler Verges designed the book cover and Insight Graphics prepared it for the printer.

I wish you well,
Leslie Dawson

Introduction

Diabetes and Your Pocketbook

To manage your diabetes, you must make choices to meet your special needs in the areas of
- Medications
- Supplies and equipment
- Food
- Exercise
- Stress
- Medical services

Within each category, you have choices. Some will cost more, others less. Some choices will make more sense to you than others, despite cost. This book is designed to help you make sensible choices in the interest of your best health. One indispensable tool in making good diabetes decisions is the telephone. Comparison shopping is much easier—and can be cheaper—when you call before you go. If you are on a budget, you are not alone in your struggle to manage diabetes. Fortunately, many government programs offer assistance for medical care, drugs, food, and other needs. Help is also available from nonprofit groups, professional organizations, and drug manufacturers.

Where are these resources? This book will help you find them. You *can* match pocketbook realities with good, safe diabetes management. Good luck and good health!$

1

Medication and Supplies

Most people with diabetes require medication. If you have type I (insulin-dependent) diabetes, you must have insulin. If you have type II (non-insulin-dependent) diabetes, you may require oral agents and/or insulin. We cannot choose to go without medication, but we can make choices to keep the total cost of medication down.

$ $ $ $ $ $ $

Medications

Insulin. Be aware that new regular insulins on the market will have much faster response times than the regular insulin you may be used to. Do not change the type of insulin (regular, lente, ultralente, or NPH) without your health-care team's advice. These insulins act very differently from one another.

Many states do not require prescriptions for insulin. However, you will need a prescription to get insulin on a drug card or to be reimbursed by your insurance company. Do comparison shopping by phone to find the best insulin prices.

Oral diabetes drugs. Oral diabetes drugs are for people with type II diabetes. Discuss your options and the costs with your doctor, and then comparison shop by phone. You may be able to obtain oral diabetes drugs at some community free clinics, municipal drug programs,

TIP: If you become homeless or very poor, your meals may be irregular or uncertain. Work out the best insulin regimen you can. Some health-care professionals recommend taking regular insulin just before meals—whenever they come. That way, you won't be caught with a high insulin level and no sugar in your blood for it to act on. Others recommend taking lente—with its slow, steady release into your system—once a day.

and other sources (see page 38).

Keep an eye on the health section of your local paper or on diabetes magazines. Once in a while you'll see an ad asking for volunteers in a diabetes research project. If you are qualified for the project, you could receive free medications for a while.

Attend free health fairs whenever you can. Sometimes diabetes-supply items are available free as well as blood testing and other health services.

High blood pressure drugs. Blood pressure control is critical to good health, especially if you have diabetes. Health-care professionals worry about low-income diabetes patients with high blood pressure. These patients often forget or ignore high blood pressure (antihypertension) drugs—even though they remember to take their diabetes medications.

Birth control drugs. Planned Parenthood offers family planning assistance, including education, no matter what your income. Birth control drugs are offered according to income, or they are free. Be sure to tell the doctor that you have diabetes. (see Resources, page 78.)

$ $ $ $ $ $ $

Shopping Around for Medications
Chain savings. Check the big guys first: drugstore chains, grocery store pharmacy chains, and pharmacies

in large retail outlets such as K-Mart. These large companies buy in such huge quantities that their prices are generally the lowest.

Independent savings. Many independent pharmacies have joined drugstore wholesale buying clubs to offer price cuts to you. Their prices may be competitive with the larger chain stores.

By telephone. Make a list of all the drugs you use, then call around and ask for the total price of your "medication package." One pharmacy or mail-order vendor may offer cut-rate insulin, but its cholesterol medication may cost more. Pick the vendor with the lowest total cost for the whole package. This method provides a safety net—the company's pharmacist knows about all the drugs you're taking. He or she can warn you about unexpected drug interactions.

Pharmacy cards. If you have health insurance that offers a pharmacy card, get one. With most cards, you pay a smaller co-pay for each prescription ($5 or $10). Other insurance plans may also require you to pay a yearly deductible plus a larger co-payment. With drug cards, you don't have to comparison shop.

Some drug coverage requires you to save receipts to submit with claim forms. It's well worth the paperwork to save those receipts. You can save up a few receipts and submit them all at once to reduce the paperwork. If you are on a tight budget, however, submit your claim as soon as you buy the medication.

Most pharmacies are now computerized. You can get a printout of your purchases for the month, year, or whatever you need.

Prescription and nonprescription drugs (such as insulin, in many states) are tax deductible. Save all receipts, and use them

> TIP: Don't save up drug receipts for the end of the year. If you wait until December, it can take a very long time to be reimbursed.

when you calculate your income tax returns.

Generic drugs. Ask your doctor to prescribe generic drugs, if possible. These copycat drugs are nearly identical to brand-name drugs. Because the patent has expired, they cost far less—some a half to a third less—than the brand-name drug. New drugs have no generic versions until their patents expire.

Bulk rates. Many pharmacists offer a discount price for larger prescriptions. Safeway pharmacies, for instance, give a cut rate for more than 100 pills for people who pay out of pocket (not for those who just pay the co-pay). Ask your pharmacist how to get the best deal, and then ask your doctor to write the prescription for that amount.

> TIP: Some insurance plans will limit subscribers to 1 month's prescription or 100 pills. Again, ask your doctor to write a prescription for the best deal. After it is filled, check to be sure you have the right prescription.

Consider travel. Some neighborhood pharmacies are just more expensive than others. Don't be surprised if inner-city drugstores charge more than outlying or suburban stores. Downtown, inner city, and crime-ridden stores pass on their higher insurance and real estate costs. (Fortunately, some large chains or supermarket pharmacies have adopted uniform pricing in all their stores.) Call to compare your neighborhood store's costs with others, especially if you have transportation to get to the distant stores to shop.

By mail-order. Compare prices among mail-order pharmacies. Some serve Medicare users only or people with insurance; others do not serve Medicare. Some sell prescription drugs; others sell supplies only. Toll-free 800 numbers for some mail-order houses are listed in the Resources chapter. A current copy of *Diabetes Forecast* has a mail-order diabetes supplies section.

Mail-order suppliers. Mail-order suppliers allow

long-distance comparison shopping. This is especially helpful for people who are housebound or who live in remote rural areas. All it takes is a phone call (they have toll-free 800 numbers) or a postage stamp.

Mail-order houses can buy in large quantities at better prices. They pass on discounts from their bulk purchases of drugs and diabetes supplies. They offer customers the best discounts for more common drugs. For new or more expensive drugs, however, mail-order prices are close to the full price. One mail-order house salesman told us that about half their drugs are at discount prices, and the others are at standard prices. (This is another good reason to compare the total cost of your medication package rather than just one or two drugs. Ask each mail-order house to give you the prices of all your drugs. Then compare the totals among all your "bidders.")

Some mail-order services specialize in nonprescription items, such as blood glucose strips, monitors, and syringes. See chapter 5 on monitoring costs.

You may not be able to use all mail-order houses—many require you to have insurance or Medicare or to use credit cards. Only a few, like AARP, will bill you.

> TIP: A lot of insurance companies offer a 3-month supply of prescriptions through mail order for a very low price. Your doctor must order the exact amount needed for 3 months and check for 3 refills.

Customer support. Before choosing a mail-order house, ask if you can use the 800 number to talk to a pharmacist—not just salespeople—when you have problems or questions. This is important. The big advantage of your local pharmacy is the pharmacist who can answer questions and watch out for possible drug interactions. He or she knows something about you, your finances, and your medical history. A pharmacist's advice is especially helpful if you are trying new drugs or new nonprescription products. Of course, if you have an unexpected reaction, call your doctor.

American Association of Retired Persons (AARP). AARP is a nonprofit association that allows nonmembers to use its mail-order pharmacy services. If you are uninsured, ask the AARP service to price your medication package. Compare its prices with your other "bids." AARP, unlike many other mail-order services, will bill you instead of asking for up-front payment. (Most mail-order houses require insurance, prepayment, or credit cards.) Call AARP at (800) 456-2277 for information about the pharmacy program.

The 800 number. Use toll-free 800 numbers for questions, comparison shopping, and placing orders. Ask for the 1-month cost of your drugs. Some mail-order services require customers to buy 3-month supplies. This is another cost saver. Make sure your doctor understands how much you order so he or she can write your prescription for the proper amount.

If your order is unexpectedly delayed, call the 800 number. The customer service department can check your order and sometimes send an emergency supply by express delivery. If they caused the delay, make sure they will also pay the added delivery cost.

Ordering prescriptions. To fill your order and arrange for insurance payment, **most mail-order houses need:**

✔The original copy of your prescription, which you must mail to them.

✔Confirmation of your good standing with your insurance company. They will contact the insurance company after you give them its name, your group identification (employer, association, or code) number, account number, and the dates for your policy's start and expiration. This information will be on your insurance card.

✔Time to fill the prescription. Allow 2–3 weeks to

receive your first order. Meanwhile, ask your physician to write two prescriptions: one to buy the drugs you need until the mail order arrives and another to send to the mail-order house. Find out what insurance or Medicare/Medicaid information the company needs before you ask your doctor to write the prescription.

$ $ $ $ $ $ $

Cutting the Costs of Nonprescription Supplies

Diabetes is the "hardware disease." Patients use computerized glucose monitors, testing strips, lancets, syringes, glucose tablets, and alcohol swabs. All these nonprescription diabetes supplies add to the high-cost burden of diabetes health care.

The average person with diabetes spends $2,500 a year in drugstores—far more than the rest of the population. The same people tend to spend most of their drugstore dollars in the same pharmacy. However, pharmacies are not necessarily the cheapest places to buy hardware. With a little shopping around, you can save money.

Blood glucose testing is like everything else. You get what you pay for. The fewer tests you make, the less helpful the information you have. Result? More guessing about mealtime calories, before-exercise food, bedtime snacks, and insulin dosages. More swings in your blood sugar. This is not healthy for you. If you want to cut back on tests for budget reasons, check with your health-care team. Bring in your glucose test records to find out when it's most important for you to test.

Test-strip savings. Blood glucose self-testing gives you information you must have to control your diabetes. However, strips range in price from 35 to 98 cents apiece. The price of testing four times a day can rise to more than $1,000 a year, which may stop you from testing very often.

✔Compare prices from large retailers, chain pharmacies, and mail-order firms. In general, large firms can buy wholesale more cheaply and pass those savings on to you.

✔Check prices with independent pharmacies belonging to buyers' clubs. Ask pharmacists at smaller drugstores if they belong to such a club. They can pass their wholesale savings on to the customer.

✔Buy in bulk. Strips come in boxes of 50 and 100. Usually, the 100-strip boxes cost a little less per strip than the 50-strip boxes. For instance, 50 strips might cost $35.99 or 72 cents per strip. The same brand of 100s might cost $66.50, or 66 cents per strip. At four tests a day, over a year you would save about $85 a year by buying 100-strip packages.

✔Consider off-brand or private label, or generic strips. Many big retailers, such as K-Mart, have house brand strips for some monitors.

Note that some diabetes educators have reported that patients using generic strips sometimes have erratic readings. Research shows mixed results. Use the test solution provided by your monitor manufacturer to check the accuracy of any strips you use. Test each new box of strips. If you find a batch of strips with unusual results, report the problem to the manufacturer (the 800 number is listed on the package). They will send you a new package of strips in exchange for the problem product. Then they can analyze what went wrong.

✔**If you buy generic strips read the package to be sure the strips can be used with your brand of monitor.** Currently, generic companies make chemical-action strips, rather than electronic-action strips. Generic products cannot be used with ExacTech or MediSense monitors.

✔Consider dividing strips lengthwise for visual readings if your doctor or educator thinks you could still get accurate readings. Although the manufacturers do not recommend it, some people do split their strips to get two for the price of one. *Caution:* **There are two types of strips.** Visual-read strips rely on a chemical/color reaction on the patch; they can be split. Electronic strips rely on an electronic reaction that runs down the strip; they cannot be split. Only split those strips with color patches.

> TIP: Check the expiration date on the test solution. Once you open the bottle, it will only be good for 3–6 months. Check the paper inside the package for the number of months. Write that expiration date on the bottle.

✔Test at critical times only. If you can't afford testing four times a day, test in the morning before breakfast and before your last insulin injection of the day. The third choice is before bed, to prevent low blood sugar reactions during the night or early morning. Test at other times if you have other patterns of lows or highs or test once a day at a different time each day.

Some other cost-savers are:

✔You don't have to swab fingerstick sites with alcohol. Cleaning well with soap and water is all you need to do.

✔Recycle lancets. You can reuse lancets for fingersticks if you leave them in the fingerstick device. Keep them in a safe place or container so other people do not get stuck.

✔Strip supply emergencies? Call the manufacturer of your monitor. Use the 800 number on the machine. Ask if any coupons or short-dated strips are avail-

> TIP: Do not split strips if you have limited dexterity or sight problems. If you have trouble reading the color of whole strips, splitting is not for you. If you do split strips, cut only one strip at a time. Be sure to put the unused split strip back into their moisture-proof container after cutting.

able for medically indigent people. Sometimes manufacturers give away strips that have used up their shelf life and can't be shipped to pharmacies.

✔Ask your diabetes educator. Many receive free samples of strips from manufacturers for helping low-income patients.

Monitor know-how. Before buying a monitor, check with your diabetes educator about which monitors are best for you. Phone around for prices in pharmacy chains, grocery

> TIP: Don't wipe strips with cotton you've saved from vitamin or medicine bottles. You'll get inaccurate results.

store pharmacies, independent pharmacies, and mail-order companies. Get copies of the latest consumer diabetes magazines (such as *Diabetes Forecast*). Remember to check your local library, your diabetes educator's office, or the local American Diabetes Association (ADA) affiliate to look at these magazines if you can't afford to buy them. Read the ads. As you ask around, check for several things:

✔Monitor cost after the rebate, and how long will it take to get that rebate?

✔Services with the monitor: Is there a toll-free 800 number you can use for questions or problems (and keep your phone bill down)? Do they provide help free of charge?

✔Strip prices: How do they compare with other strip prices? What will your monthly cost be? (Number of tests per day × price per strip × 30 days)

✔Replacement: Does the company replace monitors free when they break down? Some do, some don't.

✔Batteries: How much do the batteries cost and how long will they last? (Ask how many tests you can do on one battery and figure out how long it will last you.)

Call the company's 800 number if you have any

questions. See Resources for a list of different manufacturers. Once you have a glucose monitor, it will
probably last a long time.

If you get a meter readout that you don't trust,
check your owner's manual. If you are worried about
accuracy, check your monitor's results with the glucose
test solution made for your meter. You can also call the
monitor company's 800 number. They will help you
diagnose problems. They may send you a glucose solution to test how well your machine is working. If they
agree your machine is broken, some companies will
exchange it for a new one. Others send rebate coupons
for you to buy a replacement monitor.

Syringes: getting to the point. To save money, we
suggest the following:

✔Coupons: Use manufacturer's coupons when
they are available.

✔Private label and off brands: Ask your pharmacist about house-brand syringes. One of the major hospital supply syringe manufacturers will begin selling
private-label syringes in the summer of 1995. They
promise 30% lower prices than even their own brand-
name syringes.

✔Alcohol swabs: You don't need them. Needles
don't carry enough germs below the skin to cause
infections. Just clean your skin with soap and water.

✔Syringe recycling: You can use your syringes
more than once. If you plan to reuse, be sure to recap
the syringe after each use to protect the point. Some
people reuse syringes until the point gets dull or slightly painful to use. Others use a new syringe each day. It
all depends on your comfort level and your budget. Do
not wipe the needle with alcohol. This removes the
coating that makes the injections less painful.

Some 40–50 U.S. cities have needle-exchange programs for AIDS prevention. When you give them your
used syringe, they give you a new one. These programs

serve people tempted to share needles with others who are most at risk for AIDS. Rather than share syringes, call your municipal AIDS control department or public health department (found in the blue pages). Find out where and when needle-exchange programs take place. There,

> Never share syringes: Do not share your syringe with anyone else to save money, even in the same family. You run the risk of also sharing acquired immunodeficiency syndrome (AIDS), hepatitis, and infections.

you can exchange your used needle for a new one—no questions asked, no charge. *Caution:* Needle-exchange programs usually operate just a few times per week and sometimes in "rough" neighborhoods. Of course, you would not use this program unless you could not afford to buy any new syringes of your own.

Insulin pumps: too much for most low incomes. Although insulin pumps are an effective alternative to daily injections, they may be too expensive for people with low incomes. The pump costs $3,000–5,000. Training to use the pump can be costly, especially if the training takes place in a hospital, where you also have to pay for a few days of hospital care. Pump use requires frequent blood glucose testing. Users test four, six, or even more times a day, so testing costs are high. Whereas some insurance programs pay for pumps, Medicare does not, at the time of this writing. $

2

Frugal Foods: Eating on a Budget

In this chapter, we show you how smart shopping and simple cooking will help you eat well on a budget.

$ $ $ $ $ $ $

Dietitians and Dollars

Diabetes books all say, "Consult with a dietitian." It's good advice. Dietitians can help you combine nutrition with your daily life, your exercise patterns, and your practical limitations. Dietitians help you learn how to fit foods you like into your diet *and* your budget.

> **TIP:** Dietitians are professionals. A brief consultation costs $45–$85. If you are not covered by insurance for dietitian services, check with your local public health clinic or community free clinic. More than half of the country's local health departments employ a full- or part-time nutritionist or dietitian.

$ $ $ $ $ $ $

Food and Dollars

Eating healthy foods *does not* cost more. It's just a matter of smart choices and good timing. Here are a few tips for making smart choices.

Before You Shop

✔Does your neighborhood store have a wide food selection? Is it expensive? Have you compared these prices to other stores? Is the produce fresh—or stale and limp? Does the store offer bargains and coupons for junk food but not fresh food? You may need to shop somewhere else. If you can't, buy frozen fruits and vegetables rather than wilted produce.

✔Plan your menus. See what you already have on hand, then make a list to take to the store. Don't buy anything that is not on the list, within reason. If you had planned on apples, but grapes are on sale, take the better buy. This will keep you from wasting money on impulse buying.

✔Look for a nearby day-old-bread store. Pick whole-grain breads. Be careful though—not everything is a bargain. Buy low-fat baked goods such as bagels, tortillas, English muffins, and pita bread. Avoid high-fat crackers, doughnuts, cakes, cookies, and pastries. They aren't good for you, and they're expensive to boot!

✔Grow your own food. Use your backyard, your windowsill, or your balcony to grow vegetables. Homegrown tomatoes, peppers, and herbs will enhance your meals and pocketbook. Bonus: Gardening is a stress buster and a calorie burner.

✔Look for "pick-your-own" farms and farmers' markets in your area. Some advertise in the newspaper classified ads or the food section. The food is fresh, the cost is usually low, and you get some fresh air and exercise, too. When they have too much, some farms will give away crops such as greens.

✔Put family hunters and fishers to work. You can stock your freezer for the cost of a license. Squirrel, rabbit, dove, and venison are low-fat red meats. All kinds of fish are good for you. Bonus: Fishing and hunting are stress busters, too.

Shopping Tips

If you take the time and get organized, you can save a lot of money at the grocery store by using coupons.

Check your newspaper for coupons and ad circulars that come in the mail. Check for store coupons at the store. If your store has a savings club or special coupons for people who get a check-cashing card at the store, you should get one. It costs nothing for the card. Some stores have certain days when they give you double the amount on your coupon. These are the days to shop.

✔Join a food co-op. You get near wholesale prices for grains, beans, and foods in bulk.

✔Try not to go grocery shopping when you are hungry. You'll spend more.

✔Look for bargains on foods from all the different food groups:
- Grains, dried beans and peas, and starchy vegetables
- Fruits
- Vegetables
- Meat or Meat Substitutes
- Fats
- Milk

✔Pick up snacks for low blood sugar reactions (sugar or sugar cubes, orange juice, graham crackers, or hard candies for when you are away from home).

✔Don't buy special "diabetic" or "dietetic" foods. These may be convenient, but they're also expensive. You can eat healthy with regular foods at regular prices.

✔Pay for food, not packaging or processing. Look for brightly colored, crisp, unbruised fruits and vegetables and whole grains like rice or oatmeal. If the foods are old or wilted, choose frozen varieties.

✔Buy healthy snacks. Buy fresh fruit and vegetables, low-fat milk, or low-fat or nonfat yogurt, instead of sweets, soda, or high-fat foods. Use low-fat whole-grain crackers or bread. High-fiber foods, such as strawberries or graham crackers, cost less and are filling and satisfying.

✔Buy produce for just a few days at a time and only as much as is needed for your menus. Stored for longer periods, produce may spoil and lose nutritional value.

✔Avoid junk food. High-fat foods such as potato chips and pork rinds provide "comfort value." However, they can damage your heart—and your pocketbook.

✔Buy low-fat dairy products. Low-fat (skim or 1%) milk is healthier. Also use low-fat or nonfat yogurt, and 1% or nonfat cottage cheese. Keep nonfat dry milk powder on hand. Mix it with water and then mix it half and half with 1% milk to save money. Use it to make your own yogurt and for baking. Store opened packages in the refrigerator but don't keep them too long.

✔Buy "healthier" fats. Use vegetable (canola or olive) oils instead of animal fats (e.g., butter, bacon fat, or lard). Vegetable oils are healthier than most margarines.

✔Look for low-cost fish. Buy tuna, salmon, and sardines canned in water, tomato sauce, or mustard. Ask at the grocery store's fish department for fish scraps. They'll be free or very cheap. Gourmet cooks use these to make wonderful chowders and soups, and so can you.

✔Look for house brands. Save money and get nearly the same quality as name brands. All large grocery store chains have their own brands.

✔Limit purchases of alcohol, sweets, and fats. They are expensive choices for both your health and your pocketbook.

Food Preparation

✔Eat meals at the same times each day.

✔Cook your own meals and save money. If you work, cook ahead on weekends and freeze the dishes, or use a slow-cooker. You can make nutritious and inexpensive bean dishes, soups, and stews with brown rice, millet, wheat, or beans. Grains are inexpensive if you buy them in bulk from health food stores, grocery stores, or co-ops.

✔Refrigerate or freeze dishes in correct serving sizes for your meal plan. This saves you time and energy during the week. Freezer bags take up very little space. Label with date and content.

✔Cook your own oatmeal or mixed-grain hot cereal—it takes 5 minutes and costs much less than packaged dry cereals. If you buy in bulk, it's even cheaper.

✔Make your own skim milk yogurt. Heat your oven to 300°F. Turn the oven off. Fill a one-quart jar three-quarters full with very warm tap water, stir in 1 cup of skim milk powder, and add 1 cup yogurt. (Save a bit of yogurt from a package that says "active or live culture.") Screw on the lid, shake it all up, and wrap in two towels or several sheets of newspaper. Put in the oven (be sure it is turned off), and leave overnight. (You could also set the jar on a heating pad on low for 4 hours.) You'll have yogurt in the morning. Enjoy it with fresh fruit, cereal, applesauce, baked potatoes, or to make salad dressings. You can also make yogurt in thermos bottles. Preheat the bottles by rinsing the inside with hot water. Then pour in the milk-yogurt mixture, cap tightly, and let sit overnight.

$ $ $ $ $ $ $

Plant-Based Diet

The problem with American diets is fat. We get most of our fat from meat and milk products. One simple way to take the animal fat out of our meals is to become a vegetarian. Get help from a dietitian to do this.

Vegetarians tend not to be overweight. They have lower death rates from heart and circulatory disease and may also have less colon and breast cancer. They even have lower rates of type II diabetes. However, most people are not total vegetarians. It's cheaper and still healthy if some animal products are included in your meals.

An excellent vegetarian cookbook, with money-saving tips, is *Laurel's Kitchen*, by Laurel Robertson, Carol Flinders, and Bronwen Godfrey. You can find it in the public library or at the bookstore.

The other advantage of beans, grains, and vegetables is that they cost less than meats. If you do the cooking, you may find that your food costs actually go down. Vegetarian diets don't call for many processed foods. Fresh basic foods, cooked at home, have always been the way to save money. Consult a dietitian to be sure you're getting the right nutrients and appropriate amounts every day.

Another long-term payoff could be weight loss. You'll probably save on medical costs in the long run, too, but it's hard to figure those savings into a monthly budget. Do not attempt to go vegetarian without a good cookbook (check in your local library) and some guidelines from a dietitian.

$ $ $ $ $ $ $

Food Labels

Two kinds of labels can help you make good food choices. Labels on the shelves in the store tell you the total cost and the unit cost for each product. Compare the unit costs of different brands to get the best buy for your money.

Labels on food products tell you what is inside—serving size must be checked in relation to calories, fat, protein, and carbohydrate. Because your blood sugar is mostly affected by the carbohydrate (starch and sugar) that you eat, you may get better control of your diabetes if you count how much carbohydrate you eat at each meal and snack. A dietitian can help you learn how to do this. Carbohydrates are found in starches, grains, milk products, fruits, and vegetables. Also check the label to see if sugar or saturated fats have been added to the product in processing.

$ $ $ $ $ $ $

Supplements: Vitamins and Minerals

In general, if you eat healthy foods, you don't need vitamin or mineral supplements. If you don't eat healthy all the time, you can take a multivitamin. Ask your pharmacist for a good, low-cost supplement with minerals at 100% of the USRDA.

$ $ $ $ $ $ $

Eating Out

You probably eat out now and then. Americans spend 43% of their food budget on restaurant food. Cook at home to save money. Otherwise, here are some ways to save money!

✔Try breakfast. It may be your best buy. You may get more nutrition per dollar at breakfast than any other time. Try breakfast at an inexpensive full-service restaurant. Most have a breakfast special that includes many of the foods you need. Milk and egg dishes provide protein, plus you get important carbohydrates in cereal, toast, and potatoes. A vegetable omelet offers protein laced with carbohydrates. Ask for low-fat or skim milk with your cereal and cut more fat by choosing boiled or poached eggs. If you have high cholesterol, limit eggs, sausages, and bacon. And see if fruit or juice is included in the special.

✔Ask if the restaurant has a "nutrition facts" list on the menu. Some calculate food exchanges for you, but beware—these may change with a different cook or a smaller or larger portion.

✔Look for menu items marked "low calorie," "low-fat," or "light." Read carefully. Some are really "light," some aren't. Some places charge more for the "diet" plate. The main dishes will probably suit you just as well.

✔Choose broiled chicken or a small hamburger. Avoid deep-fried chicken or fish.

✔Use the salad bar. Salad can be a whole meal if it includes cottage cheese and beans for protein. Avoid the heavy salad dressings. If you hate the "lite" salad dressings, mix your own with vinegar, a little oil, salt, and pepper, or take a nonfat dressing with you.

✔Order skim or 1% milk or fruit juice. For the same price, these provide more food value than soda, coffee, or tea. If there are unlimited refills of the tea, it has healthy antioxidants to recommend it as a good choice.

✔Dine ethnic. You can find inexpensive nutritious meals in many ethnic restaurants. They often serve unfried food, nonmeat proteins, and tasty vegetable dishes at low prices.

Chinese. Cheap lunch specials usually include meat, vegetables, and rice. Check out the "mein" dishes— bowls of noodles with chopped meats and vegetables— or the tofu dishes. Watch out for fried dishes or other methods that add fat.

Mexican. Soft tacos or burritos with beans or chicken are a good nutritious buy. Avoid deep-fried dishes such as chimichangas.

Italian. A basic pasta dish is hard to beat for the price. Pizza is an important part of American diets. Unfortunately, pizza is high in calories and fat and can cause rapid rises in blood glucose for 4–9 hours after the meal. Test to see how pizza affects you.

Middle Eastern and Indian. Look for specials that combine kebabs, yogurt/cucumber salad, vegetables, and rice.

$ $ $ $ $ $ $

When the Cupboard's Bare

Sometimes we find ourselves with nothing to eat. That's the time to check out government food assistance, food banks, churches, soup kitchens, and other charities. If your problem is a long-term situation, apply for government food assistance. Several programs are available:

Food stamps. For low-income individuals or families.

WIC (Women, Infants, and Children). For low-income women (pregnant and new mothers), and their infants and children.

Meals-on-wheels. For homebound, low-income people, those who are 65 years of age or older, or those who are disabled.

Surplus foods. Free foods for low-income people. (see Chapter 7 for more information.)

Search your community for more immediate food assistance—a food bank or soup kitchen. Your local public assistance office may help you find one. Or, look in the Yellow Pages under "social service organizations." This listing includes both government and charitable groups. Call an umbrella group such as United Way, Catholic Charities, The Salvation Army, or one of the hot lines listed in the phone book.

Some people feel too shy or too proud to ask for charity. You might feel better by promising yourself to give back your first spare dollar to the soup kitchen or vowing to join these workers as a volunteer when you can.

$ $ $ $ $ $ $

Homelessness

If you should become homeless, find out the locations and schedules for homeless shelter meals—and **when** to line up. Look in the Yellow Pages under "social service organizations," as discussed above.

21

Soup kitchens offer nutritious meals. Find out their schedules. Once you have a reliable meal schedule, you can work out with your doctor an insulin or oral-agent regimen to go with it.

✔Ask shelter staff people if you may have a sandwich to prevent low-blood sugar reactions during the day. Do not assume that they understand diabetes. Explain your diabetes and that you must have midday food to prevent low blood sugars.

✔Don't settle for bakery goods and coffee in the morning. Now is when you need the best fuel for your body. Try to get a teaspoon or more of fat and some protein in the morning. A small serving of meat, cheese, or peanut butter will help keep you going all day.

✔Hide syringes and pills from people in the shelter or on the street. Drug users sometimes steal syringes and pills.

✔Wear an identification (ID) bracelet. The stresses of homelessness put you at high risk of a diabetic crisis. If you become unconscious, an ID bracelet calls out for the right kind of help—fast.

✔Check your feet *every* day. Homeless people can spend hours walking and standing in line daily. Feet often become swollen and ulcerated. Check your feet daily, and if you find a problem, seek medical help immediately. Without medical help, a small sore could result in gangrene, amputation, or even death. It's worthwhile to try to find a comfortable pair of athletic shoes or boots at a nearby thrift store. Never walk around barefooted. $

3

Low-Expense Exercise

Regular exercise is the cheapest part of good diabetes management. It's free. Did you know that exercise helps insulin move into your cells and that exercise affects blood glucose levels for hours after you finish? Regular exercise does help your body use insulin and blood glucose more efficiently, which means you may get to cut back on the amount of insulin or pills you take. This may save you money.

You don't have to huff and puff. Go at your own pace. Exercising for half an hour or more one or two hours after a meal has the greatest effect. When you stimulate your heart and lungs by moving, you're healthier. Plus, exercise helps you lose weight better than dieting alone. In fact, you may not need to diet if you add exercise to your lifestyle. Exercise rebuilds the muscle that you lose with the passing years. You want muscles because they help you lose weight. Muscles that have been worked keep burning calories even when they are at rest.

No Excuses

Your neighborhood's not safe? See if a nearby shopping center or senior center has a walking group. If they don't, start one. Get permission to walk before mall stores open or get some friends together and form a walking "posse." Kill two birds with one stone—neighborhood safety and exercise. You don't get outdoors? Turn on a television exercise program or video. You can borrow exercise videos and books from the public library. To keep yourself going, exercise with a friend.

Before You Start

Start any exercise program slowly, checking out how your blood sugar and your heart rate respond. Check with your health-care team before you start any new activity. Ask about special precautions you should take if you have:

✔**Heart and circulation problems**. Ask what heart rates are safe for you. Learn how to check your pulse to see how hard you are working.

✔**Eye problems**. For some eye conditions, you must avoid jolts, high-impact activities, or bending over so that blood rushes to your head. Ask your health-care team for safe exercises for you.

✔**Foot problems**. Check with your health-care team. You may not be able to run or walk if you have foot ulcers or get bone fractures easily. You may need

> **TIP:** Always shop for shoes late in the day, when your feet may be more swollen than in the morning. You want your shoes to fit all day.

therapeutic shoes (prescription shoes, or nonprescription "comfort" shoes) or a well-fitted pair of athletic shoes. Some therapeutic shoe stores have sale racks with expensive, comfortable shoes at a bargain price. (See chapter 7 on Medicare coverage for therapeutic shoes.) Always wear clean, well-fitting socks.

✔**Nerve damage**. Do you have diabetic nerve damage, i.e., neuropathy? Check with your health-care team. They will proba-

> **TIP:** Sometimes a $20 insole purchased at a sport shoe store is enough to turn your shoes into "expensive" comfort shoes!

24

bly recommend that you exercise only up to a moderate level, because you may not be able to feel pain when a part of your body is working too hard. For instance, you may not be able to feel if your heart is beating too fast or if you are developing a blister on your foot.

✔**Drugs**. Check with your health-care team to see how exercise and the drugs you are taking will affect you. For example, some high blood pressure drugs slow down your heart rate. If you're not sure how exercise and your drugs are going to affect your blood sugar levels, you may need to test during and after exercise for a while.

OK, Let's Do It

Ideally, you should exercise for 30–45 minutes a day, 3–5 days a week. You'll do it if you choose one or two activities that you really like to do.

If you do physical work on the job, try other types of exercise at home. For example, if you do lots of lifting at work, walk or jog. If you stand a lot, lie down and get those feet above your heart. Your ankles will thank you. Whatever your activity, remember to finish with some stretching. Stretching makes you flexibile and strong, and it feels good. Always check with your doctor first about the level of exercise best for you.

Here are some low-cost workout suggestions. They don't require special equipment or gym fees:

✔**Light exercise.** If you've never exercised or haven't in a long time, begin slowly. Try gentle stretching and slow walking. Or, double the benefits—turn on some dance music and slow dance with your honey for half an hour. You can dance alone, too. Exercise programs for older people or those with disabilities may involve sitting in a hard-backed chair and stretching. Use two soup cans for weights during arm raises. Hold two scarves and wave them up, down, around, and back to the music. (See Resources for the 800 number for Armchair Fitness Videos.)

✔**Moderate exercise.**
Try faster walking, slow
jogging, walking up stairs,
walking in the pool, or vig-
orous housework. Find a

> **TIP:** Make music part
> of your workout. Music
> helps you pace your-
> self and is relaxing.

video or TV aerobics program that fits your fitness
level. Or, grab your honey again and dance to fast
music. *Caution:* If you have diabetic eye problems,
check with your doctor.

✔**Heavy exercise.** Try running up the stairs, jump-
ing rope, chopping wood in the backyard, or competing
in local 5K and 10K races. (See *Caution* above.)

✔**Swimming.** Swimming is easy on your joints
and a great allover workout. Use a board for kicking to
build up your stamina. Your community pool may cost
a dollar for a swim. Find out whether you can save
money with special passes for a whole season or many
visits. Ask when you can do lap swimming or join special groups, such as "master" (middle-aged or older)
swimmers.

> **TIP:** Video workouts are fun, because they provide
> music and a variety of exercises in the privacy of
> your home. Rent or borrow workout videos at video
> stores, grocery stores, or the library. Read the label
> to find a routine that matches your level of fitness.

Exercise Guidelines

✔Never exercise when your blood sugar is over
250 mg/dl and your urine has ketones in it.

✔Exercise 3–5 sessions per week. (Five sessions
works best for weight loss.)

✔Each session should last 20–60 minutes.

✔Exercise at 50–70% of your "maximum aerobic
capacity" for 20–60 minutes. That means not too hard
and not too slow. If you go slowly, then exercise for a
longer time. Ask your health-care team for help with this.

> **TIP:** Find low-cost exercise weights in your kitchen. Two 14-ounce cans of tomatoes are great for starters. Experts suggest different sizes of weights, because some muscles are stronger than others and need more work. Choose cans, ketchup bottles, etc., checking the weights on the labels. Make sure you can hold them comfortably. For leg weights, put cans or 1-, 2-, or 5-pound bags of flour in a shopping bag. Sit on a stool, put the handle over your ankle, and lift.

✔If you're working hard, your glucose reading may be higher immediately after exercise.

✔Don't exercise when the weather is very cold, very hot, or very humid.

✔Go to the library and look under "exercise." (Number 671 in library shelving code numbers.) Check in the library for videos, too.

✔Carry a fast-acting source of sugar with you during exercise in case you go low (juice, milk, hard candies, or glucose tablets.

✔If you take insulin or a diabetes pill, exercise with a friend who can help you if you go low.

✔Know where your blood sugar level is before exercise and after. Then you'll know if you need a snack to get you through it.

✔Work with your doctor to adjust your medication to your exercise program once it becomes regular.

After exercise, stretch like a cat, feeling all your muscles, slow . . . easy . . . and relax. Say good-bye to stress.

If someone's handy, ask for a nice back rub or a foot massage. **$**

4

Diabetes and Low Income = Stress

The word stress is used so much these days, it's almost a cliche. After all, *everybody* has stress, don't they? Well, there's stress, and then there is *stress*. Some people are surprised when "happy" stress—like a wedding—may cause the same high blood sugar that "bad" stress—like losing a job—causes. Think of stress as anything that demands a response from you. Your response to stress can range from depression to high blood sugar. That's why stress management is a high priority for everyone with diabetes.

$ $ $ $ $ $ $

Stress Will Mess With Glucose Levels
Blood glucose goes up and down when you're under stress. Here are some reasons why.

✔Depression can alter blood sugar levels.

✔Stress makes some people "insulin resistant." Even when insulin is in your blood, your body cells can't use it well. Then your blood sugar levels go up.

✔Stress can make it harder to stick to your diet, exercise, and medication regimen.

✔Stress directly affects some diabetes complications. High blood pressure (hypertension) is very sensitive to stress. Long-term high blood pressure can make other complications (such as kidney disease and heart disease) worse.

✔The stress of diabetes pushes some people into eating disorders (anorexia and bulimia) and depression. Eating disorders involve vomiting, refusing to eat, and binging. These behaviors make it harder for you to get nutrients and to keep blood-sugar levels stable. They also interfere with your exercise schedule. Depression can either increase or decrease your appetite, cause excessive sleepiness, and create other problems. Again, your diabetes self-care plan can go out the window.

Causes of Stress

✔Stress builds when you deny that you really have diabetes or need medical or psychological help.

✔Stress builds when you worry about lowered sexual performance or pleasure as a result of sexual dysfunction caused by diabetes.

✔Stress builds when diabetes lowers your self-esteem.

✔Stress may come with low income—with or without diabetes.

$ $ $ $ $ $ $

Managing Stress

So what can you do?

Make healthy choices. No matter how bad things look, you always have some choices. Learn which stresses you must handle and which you can avoid or change.

✔If your job is highly stressful, check the classifieds for other openings in your field. Maybe you don't have to stay in that job.

✔Does your brother-in-law upset you? Stop socializing with him.

✔If you have been drinking too much, go to an Alcoholics Anonymous meeting.

✔Quit smoking. It's not easy, but it's healthier and it will save you money.

✔Change your own negative behaviors or attitudes. It's easier to change yourself than somebody else.

✔You can improve your skills by going back to school.

Talk to someone. When the going gets tough, talking to someone can help. Talking to a good listener can lower your blood pressure—and your blood sugar. A good listener hears you out without pushing his or her opinions and recommendations on you. A good listener helps you get your concerns into the open, where you can consider your choices.

Ask for help. Sometimes it's too personal or your good listener is out of town. Time to get a professional listener—free. If you're nervous about asking for help, call a hot line. Look in the Yellow Pages under "crisis intervention" or "social service organizations," or just ask the information operator for a crisis hot line. Most hot lines are 24-hour services, attended by trained volunteers. They will steer you toward professionals if you need further help.

Relax the mind and body. Everybody has different ways to relax. What's yours? It could be music, reading, dancing, watching television, or getting a neck massage. Check in the library under "exercise" to find a variety of books describing stress-reducing exercises.

Exercise your body daily. Walk. Our bodies were

Cost-Free Stress Busters

• **Make an appointment with yourself:** Make time for relaxing.
• **Look at the problem from a new angle**, even if it seems silly or outrageous.
• **Join a support group:** You feel better when you have others to share your experiences.
• **Just say "no"** to demands on your energy and time.
• **Distract yourself from your troubles:** Smell the roses, watch the birds, make music, talk to a friend.

made to move. Moving quiets the mind and makes you feel better. Read the Exercise chapter and find activities that are right for you.

Exercise your spiritual resources. Research confirms what many people have known all their lives—prayer is powerful. Scientists found that people with active spiritual lives resisted and fought off depression better.

$ $ $ $ $ $ $

Depression

Depression is a medical problem if

✔You stop caring about your diabetes self-care routines,

✔You start sleeping the day away,

✔You can't get to sleep at all,

✔You are weepy all the time,

✔You feel a sense of utter despair,

✔You find yourself thinking that death or suicide is the way out.

If you are severely depressed, call for medical help. You can get immediate counseling on a crisis hot line. $

5

Health Care:
Cutting the Costs

You do have choices for health care. There are health insurance, low-cost health care, Medicare coverage (if you are over age 62 years or disabled), and some free health care.

$ $ $ $ $ $ $

Insurance

The health insurance industry essentially bets that they'll make more money on payments and interest than the customer will claim for health-care expenses. However, some companies decide that people with diabetes are poor bets. You may either be turned down for insurance or have to pay higher premiums and deductibles.

Some companies take an enlightened approach to diabetes. If you have controlled diabetes, chances are good that you can obtain low-cost, managed-care health insurance. "If diabetes is controlled, we consider the risk fairly minimal," said one health insurance underwriter. "In general, these people are in good health overall. And people with diabetes are actually more in tune with their bodies than other people. They pay much more attention to good diet and exercise."

There are two major types of health insurance:

Indemnity insurance. Traditional (indemnity) health insurance offers a choice of doctors and hospitals but often with more expensive premiums. Consumers choose their own health-care professionals. Frequently, these insurance programs make you wait 6–9 months or longer before they will pay any expenses for preexisting conditions such as diabetes.

Managed-care insurance. You'll probably have better luck and lower costs with managed health care—preferred provider organizations (PPOs), or health maintenance organizations (HMOs). They cut costs to you (and the insurance company) by

✔limiting the list of health-care providers you may see,

✔asking preferred providers and hospitals to charge set prices for services,

✔having a primary-care physician or professional "manage" your case,

✔centralizing care into large facilities and laboratories, and

✔incorporating preventive medicine—such as diabetes education—into their programs.

In many states, Medicare and Medicaid programs are being contracted out to managed-care facilities and HMOs.

No insurance, higher blood sugars. That's the sad truth. A recent study showed that low-income people with diabetes had better-controlled blood glucose if they had Medicare, Medicaid, or health insurance. Those without health coverage had higher blood sugars, as indicated by their hemoglobin (HbA_{1c}) tests. If there is any way you can get insurance, it will probably pay off in your diabetes management and your general health.

Lower-cost health insurance is becoming more available as managed-care companies and HMOs compete for customers. Some HMOs have grown so large that they are reducing the cost of their premiums. Many HMOs allow people with diabetes to participate without much fuss. Preexisting conditions, such as diabetes, are covered right away.

Shopping for insurance. Insurance plans are like everything else. There are good ones and not-so-good ones. If you are looking into an HMO or another insurance program, ask these questions:

✔What will I have to pay for premiums?

✔Are there any restrictions on preexisting conditions?

✔How long do I have to wait before my diabetes expenses are covered?

✔Will I have to pay a yearly deductible? If so, how much?

✔Are there co-payments for visits? How much?

✔Is there a pharmacy program? What's the co-payment?

✔Does the pharmacy program cover glucose testing strips, insulin, and therapeutic shoes?

✔Does the pharmacy program offer savings for generic drugs?

✔Is there a preventive health program? Does it cover
- diabetes education?
- yearly eye examinations?
- dietitians?
- exercise specialists?

✔Does the program have its own diabetes center or diabetes specialists?

✔How difficult is it to see specialists, especially
- endocrinologists?
- neurologists?
- heart and circulation specialists?
- podiatrists?
- psychiatrists or psychologists? (Is there an extra charge?)
- kidney specialists?
- others you may need?

HMOs may provide lower-cost medical care. Indemnity programs offer more choice but at a higher cost. You'll have to make compromises somewhere. Choose the program that meets most of your needs.

Keep your eyes open for insurance plans through your workplace, community hospitals, church, school, professional organizations, unions, and fraternal or social organizations. Some insurance plans take on individuals at certain times of the year—watch for their advertisements in the newspaper or on televsion. Some may request a letter from your doctor stating that you are in "good" health. Many insurance providers also ask for HbA_{1c} levels, blood pressure readings, and a list of the drugs you are taking.

> **TIP:** If you are looking for supplemental insurance for Medicare (Medigap insurance), beware of shady advertising and fraud that will get you to buy more than you need. (See Medicare in chapter 7)

$$\$\,\$\,\$\,\$\,\$\,\$\,\$$

Low-Cost and Free Health Care

Many sources of low-cost or free health care listed below require the same information about you and your financial state. When you check in, try to bring a picture ID card, such as a driver's licence, proof of your income (such as paycheck stubs or a letter from your employer), and any Medicaid/Medicare cards for you and your family members. Here are your best bets for low-cost care.

Local Public Health Departments

Most municipalities sponsor public health clinics and services. (Exceptions: Vermont, Delaware, Hawaii, and Rhode Island do not have local health departments. Public health is provided by the state.) In rural areas, public health departments may be the sole providers of health care for medically indigent people. The cost is usually on a sliding scale—the less you make, the less you pay. Most accept Medicaid, Medicare, and insured patients. Some charge no fees for services.

If you have a social worker, make sure he or she knows about your medical needs. Social workers are experts on local assistance programs, and they know how to make them work. If you check in with a public health service clinic, much of your health care will come from a registered nurse.

Municipal programs. Depending on the financial resources of the public health departments, specialized clinics may be available for:

Adult Primary Care	Immunization
Child Health	Family Planning
Dental	Gynecology
Diabetes	Emergencies
School Health	Geriatrics
Sexually Transmitted Diseases	HIV
Substance Abuse	Mental Health
Transport (for medical needs)	Tuberculosis
Pregnancy	WIC/Nutrition Services
Pharmacy	X-Rays

Flu and pneumonia vaccines. Nearly all health departments offer immunizations. Often free or low-cost flu and pneumonia vaccinations are available. People with diabetes, at risk for both these sicknesses, should take advantage of these services.

Migrant services. Certain municipalities have special clinics serving migrant workers. These clinics offer essentially similar services or are linked with other local health services.

> **TIP:** Get your flu shot in November. Waiting until the flu season starts may be too late.

General relief. Some municipalities have medical funds for people who "fall through the cracks." Take, for example, a person who has applied for Medicaid, but has not yet been approved. The patient must show this documentation to the medical clinic where he or she is seeking medical care. The county social services might allot $400 for medical expenses. Ask your social services department about general relief funds if you are awaiting approval for another program or you just don't fit into any assistance category.

Health Care for the Homeless. In more than 120 communities, federal government-funded clinics serve homeless people. In 1992, nearly 12,000 people with diabetes received help at these clinics. Call your local health department to find a clinic in your area, or call the program's national information number, (202) 628-5660.

Municipal hospitals, clinics, and emergency rooms. Many uninsured and low-income patients use municipal hospital emergency rooms for primary care. If you are sick, go there. For routine care, however, try to get into the hospital's outpatient diabetes clinic, where you will receive the specialized care you need. Municipal hospitals must serve medically indigent people, in most cases. As with all government programs, take your ID and any financial information you have.

Not-for-Profit Hospitals
Hospitals run by church and charitable organizations serve needy people as part of their mission. Here's the good news: To keep their nonprofit tax status, nonprofit hospitals must prove their charitable efforts to the government every year. They must show that they actually served the right number of medically indigent patients. Think of yourself as helping them out with this problem!

Don't feel shy about seeking medical care from a charity or religious hospital. Every year, they budget money to care for medically indigent people.

Community Free Clinics

About 155 communities are blessed with free clinics for the working poor. Doctors, nurses, and other medical professionals volunteer their time. Don't judge free clinics by their address or clientele—wait to meet the doctors and nurses serving the people. These clinics operate differently in every community, so you have to check on the hours. Some free clinics make a point of being open evening hours for working people. Call the Free Clinic Foundation in Virginia at their national number, (703) 344-8242, to find a free clinic near you, or ask your local public health department, or look in the Yellow Pages under "clinics" or "social service organizations."

Urgent Care Clinics

These private clinics are the medical equivalent of your neighborhood convenience store. You can get quick, 24-hour medical help with no appointment. They are usually more expensive than using your regular doctor but are cheaper and faster than emergency rooms.

Urgent care clinics provide care for urgent, but not emergency, problems. These clinics expect to serve a certain number of medically indigent clients every month. If you need help, call ahead, explain your situation, and ask if you can be treated.

Diabetes-Care Centers

Some diabetes clinics have limited funding to care for medically indigent people with diabetes. Call the diabetes centers in your community to find out if you can be assisted there.

Hot Lines for Diabetes, Health Care, or Mental Health

Some clinics and health services have hot lines. They are staffed with trained volunteers or medical professionals who can actually give advice, not just tell you to see a doctor. Save yourself a trip and call if you think you have a problem. Look in the Yellow Pages under "crisis intervention" or "mental health."

$ $ $ $ $ $ $

Recruiting Your Diabetes Team

To live with diabetes, you need help from a diabetes-care team—a primary-care physician or endocrinologist, diabetes nurse, and dietitian for starters. Periodically, you should see an ophthalmologist and a dentist and, for special problems, a social worker, psychologist, urologist, neurologist, or others.

The easiest way to find this health-care team is through a diabetes-care and education center. These centers have a core staff of diabetes specialist doctors, nurses, and dietitians. They have working arrangements with other specialists. It's a cost-effective, one-stop shop for diabetes care. Diabetes centers usually require that a doctor refer you.

Shopping for a Doctor

Ideally, you should see an endocrinologist, who is most likely to be current with the latest research on diabetes and its treatment. However, many primary-care doctors and internists specialize in diabetes care. If you have the luxury of choosing a doctor, ask a few questions:

✔What diabetes training does s/he have beyond basic medical school? (Doctors, nurses, and dietitians can take special seminars, become CDEs, and go to ADA and Endocrine Society professional meetings.)

✔How many of his or her patients have diabetes? (The more the better.) More with type I or type II? (Be sure it matches your diabetes.)

✔What routine tests and examinations will s/he do for diabetes? (The list should include blood sugar, HbA_{1c}, urine protein and creatinine, foot exams, and yearly dilated eye exams.)

✔Is the doctor part of a diabetes treatment team? Check whether s/he makes referrals to professionals including:

- •diabetes educator
- •eye doctor (once a year, minimum)
- •dietitian
- •podiatrist (foot doctor)
- •dentist
- •social worker or mental health professional.

Other specialists you might ask about are

- •pediatric endocrinologist (for children with diabetes)
- •nephrologist (for kidney disease)
- •neurologist (for neuropathy)
- •vascular surgeon (for circulation problems)
- •high risk obstetrician (for diabetic pregnancies)
- •gastroenterologist (for digestive problems)
- •urologist (for impotence and urinary problems).

✔Is s/he familiar with the results of the Diabetes Control and Complications Trial (DCCT)?

✔Can patients call with questions about routine diabetes care or difficulties? (Can these be discussed on the phone, or is an appointment always required?)

✔Can you use fax, modem, or mail to send in your blood-sugar records and discuss them on the phone (to reduce costs or transportation difficulties)?

Saving Dollars With a Diabetes Educator

You and your doctor need a good working relationship with a diabetes educator. Whether a nurse or a dietitian, an educator with special diabetes training can see you for less money per appointment. Nurses and dietitians with CDE after their names are certified diabetes educators and have the latest information on diabetes. Some diabetes education programs are Recognized by the American Diabetes Association as meeting the national standards for diabetes education.

Most diabetes care and education centers require you to go through an initial education program. During that time, you get to know a diabetes educator who will work with you. If you can manage it, it's worth the time and effort. If you can't afford the fee, ask the clinic if you can make special payment arrangements. They may have "scholarships" for low-income people. After the educator gets to know you, many of your routine diabetes questions and difficulties can be dealt with on the telephone. In some states, diabetes educators can also change your insulin prescriptions.

Caution: Many insurance and government programs do not cover diabetes education or nutrition services. You may have to work out a way to be sure your educator gets paid.

Alert: Watch for out-of-date diabetes professionals!
Many doctors, nurses, and dietitians think they know all about diabetes. Unfortunately, not all are up-to-date on the latest diabetes treatments. Understanding diabetes seems to be getting more complicated, not easier. Watch out for health-care professionals who:

✔do not consider type II diabetes a serious condition; **it is**.

✔blame most diabetes problems on you for not doing what you're supposed to do.

✔don't take the time to answer questions or explain something you don't understand.

✔tell you you have borderline diabetes.

If your professionals do these things, talk to them about your concerns. If they don't help you, then run, don't walk, to a different provider. Bad diabetes care will cost you in the long run.

Diabetes Support Groups
Your local ADA chapter may be able to tell you about diabetes support groups. Such a group can help you through tough times with **free**

✔education/guest speakers

✔problem-solving ideas from those who've "been there"

41

✓psychological support (amateur, of course)
✓telephone numbers to call when you need help
✓referrals to good professionals
✓laughs. (Bet you could use a few!)

$ $ $ $ $ $ $

Family-Planning Services

Birth control is especially important for women with diabetes—and their financial health. Pregnancy can be difficult for some diabetic mothers and their babies. Unplanned pregnancies can also stretch a family budget beyond its capacity.

Talk with your health-care provider before you get pregnant. Together, you can weigh the risks and benefits of pregnancy. Women with diabetes need to have their glucose levels in excellent control for 3–6 months before pregnancy to avoid complications for both mother and baby.

Many state health departments have low-cost services for pregnant women. Look in the blue pages under state listings for health and public health.

Planned Parenthood offers financial assistance for family planning. Be sure to tell the health-care professional that you have diabetes. For more information, call (800) 782-2859, to find a program near you.

Catholic Charities offers a full range of family and pregnancy counseling. Be sure to tell your health-care professional you have diabetes. Look under the white section in the telephone book for Catholic Charities or call the national number, (800) CARE-002.

$ $ $ $ $ $ $

Transportation and Medical Care

Many low-income families, especially in urban areas, do not have cars. Most of the time, mass transportation will do. There's usually a bus or a train. Sometimes mass transportation doesn't work, however—your specialist is in a distant area, or you can't take that much time off work. People in rural areas have even greater difficulties getting medical help. One study showed that people who live more than 100 miles from their clinic had the worst problems. They were most likely to drop out of diabetes treatment. To help with your transportation problems, check the following:

✔**Municipal health departments.** Yours may have a transportation program for medically indigent people. Many have one for "officially" disabled people, but not for others. Diabetes is an "official" disability.

✔**Free clinics, churches.** Volunteers may help with medical transportation.

✔**The telephone.** Sometimes, you just need to talk to the doctor or nurse. Call and explain your situation and ask if you can have a "telephone appointment."

✔**Hi-tech transport.** Some doctors and nurses are happy to receive your blood sugar records by fax or mail and then talk over the phone about them (records). Other offices have computer modems to receive information. Paying a few dollars to fax your records from a local store can save you money and time.

✔**One-stop medical shop.** Centralize all your medical services under one roof. This is the big advantage of many HMOs, hospital clinics, or group practices. It's one-stop medical shopping. Your primary physician can get your lab tests done down the hall and have a specialist look at a problem right away. You check in at the pharmacy on the way out. All for one bus fare. $

The Hemoglobin Test:
Is the HbA_{1c} Worth the Cost?

The hemoglobin test tells how your blood sugar control has been over the past 3 months. Next to doing home testing every day, it's your best measure of control.

With this test, the doctor can tell how you've been doing even if you can't do frequent blood tests yourself. **Excess glucose or sugar in your blood sticks—permanently—to a blood protein called hemoglobin.** The test measures how much gets stuck and that tells the doctor—and you—how your sugar control has been. You may be doing fine on your food, exercise, and medication schedule. This is good for you to know. If you aren't, you and your doctor can work on making changes to get your blood sugar under better control. That will keep you healthier in the long run.

The test may be offered at a free clinic near you, for the cost of a donation. The information it gives you is extremely important to your health.

6

Out of Money, Out of Medicine, Out of Food: Crisis and Illness Management

It is difficult to plan for every financial and personal crisis that can happen to you and your family. These suggestions are for emergency situations.

$ $ $ $ $ $ $

Care for Crises or Sick Days

✔Don't waste time or energy being embarrassed. Talk to your health-care provider.

✔Reduce your blood glucose testing. Cut back to morning and bedtime tests. If you can only test once a day, do it before breakfast. If you can test a few times a week, do the morning test but vary the other times to see how you're doing at different times of the day. Even three times a week will give you and your health-care team an idea of how your blood glucose control is doing.

✔It's hard to figure out what's going on unless you keep frequent records of blood glucose and ketones, and you may not be able to do that. You must call your doctor, nurse educator, dietitian, or hot line for guidance.

✔Your doctor will give you guidelines for adjusting your insulin. People with type I diabetes usually need doses of fast-acting regular insulin, even if they usually take some other type of insulin.

✔Practice stress management tools that work for you. Whether it's walking, yoga, or music, do it.

✔Be regular about meal times and what you eat at each meal. Sticking to a routine can help you when you don't have blood glucose tests to keep you on track.

Eat Lightly

Try milk or milkshakes; cereals; sandwiches; fruit and vegetable juices; cheese (American and cottage); canned soups, fruits, and vegetables; sugar-free puddings and gelatins. For salt replacement, go for canned soups, tomato juice, and cheeses. Keep canned or packaged foods for emergencies.

Drink Up

If you're sweating, vomiting, or have diarrhea, you need extra fluid. Drink a glassful of nonalcohol, noncaffeine fluid every hour. For high blood sugar periods, drink sugar-free soda, sugar-free gelatin, broth, or caffeine-free tea. For low blood sugar periods, drink regular soda, or fruit juice. If you have diarrhea or vomiting, have salty broths or a sports drink such as Gatorade.

Blood Sugars

High blood sugar. Illness or stress can cause your blood sugars to run high. Watch for symptoms such as these:

Thirst

Blurry vision

Dry mouth

Urinating more than usual

If you sense that your blood sugar is high, check if you are eating more than normal. Sometimes, people in crisis feel depressed and use snacking as "comfort food." Plus, stress alone can cause high blood sugars (see chapter 4). If you do not correct high blood sugar, it can develop into life-threatening ketoacidosis. You could go into a coma.

Ketoacidosis comes on quickly if you stop taking your insulin. Illness or stress can also cause ketoacidosis. When you are sick and cannot eat, your body calls on stored glucose, so you still need to take your insulin. The easiest way to identify ketoacidosis is to use urine-testing strips for ketones. Pay attention to these symptoms of very high blood sugar:

✔Fruity odor on breath

✔Nausea, vomiting, or abdominal pain (especially vomiting more than twice in 4 hours)

✔Difficulty breathing or rapid heartbeat

✔Difficulty paying attention, mental confusion.

Don't confuse these with flu symptoms. If you have these symptoms, plus glucose levels above 240 mg/dl and urine tests showing large ketones, **CALL YOUR DOCTOR OR GO TO THE HOSPITAL.**

Low blood sugar. Illness can also cause low blood sugar. Learn your body's signals for low blood glucose levels. These may include:

Confusion	Light-headedness
Hunger	Sweating
Sleepiness	Chills
Shakiness	Rapid heartbeat
Nausea	Irritability
Anxiety	Tingling
Strange behavior	Lack of coordination
Headaches	Stubbornness
Sadness	Delirium
Unconsciousness	Nightmares

If your symptoms or your tests indicate low blood sugar levels, take action. Drink 1/2 cup of orange juice, regular soda, or milk, or eat a light snack. Wait 15 minutes after you treat and test your blood sugar to be sure your level is up to a safe range. If it is not safe, eat again. If you do not have test strips and you do not feel better 15 minutes after treatment, eat again. If you cannot eat or drink, you may need a glucagon injection from a friend or family member. Always notify your doctor of any low blood sugar episodes because your medication may need to be adjusted.

When to Call the Doctor

Call a doctor when you have

✔Fever

✔Hypoglycemia

✔Persistent vomiting or diarrhea

✔Unusual smells in urine or vaginal discharge

✔Unexplained persistent high or low blood sugar readings

✔Day-to-day changes in your vision

✔Unusual swelling, pain, or ulcers on the legs or feet

✔Numbness in the limbs

✔Severe depression

✔Any infection or symptom that won't go away

✔Flu

✔Blood in urine, stool, or phlegm.

When to Go to the Hospital

Go to the emergency room if you have

✔Slow, shallow breathing and mental confusion,

✔Ketoacidosis, or large amounts of ketones in your urine,

✔Periods of unconsciousness from low or high blood sugar,

✔Been told by a health-care worker or hot line advisor to go.

Don't go to the emergency room with routine problems such as low-grade fever, sore throat, etc. It's *much* cheaper and faster to go to a 24-hour urgent-care center, your doctor's office, or a free clinic. (Look in the Yellow Pages under "clinics.")

$ $ $ $ $ $ $

Financial Help During Crisis

✔If it's a choice between rent, medicine, or food—call your local or state housing assistance department. Call before you pay the rent. Most communities have a housing emergency office for one-time-only situations. They may pay the rent or lend you money for 1 month's rent. Your local public assistance office may also have information on emergency housing assistance.

✔Seek emergency food stamps and food assistance if you are low on food (see chapter 7).

✔Buy smaller amounts of drugs. You don't have to buy the whole month's supply at once. You might just buy enough for a week instead.

✔When you can, save a vial of insulin or bottle of oral medication and a few glucose and ketone testing strips for hard times. Check the expiration dates, and rotate your supplies to make sure the ones you are saving don't go out of date.

✔You don't have to buy a whole vial of ketone-testing strips. Your pharmacy may sell them in packages of as few as 20 strips.

$ $ $ $ $ $ $

How to Find Crisis Pharmaceutical Help

Don't wait until all your medication is gone. For emergency assistance with prescriptions contact:

Municipal pharmacy programs. Ask your local health department (look in the blue pages of the phone book) if your city or county has a pharmacy program with medications and syringes for free or for a low co-payment. They might offer medications at a special medications clinic on certain days or at a local public or charitable hospital dispensary.

Ask the health department or the clinic if you must sign up on a different day from the day you can receive drugs. You might have to make a separate trip to do the paperwork before you can get your medication.

Diabetes clinics (hospital-associated or for-profit clinics). Some offer emergency pharmacy aid. Call local hospitals to see whether they have walk-in diabetes clinics, or look up "diabetes" in the white pages, or "clinics" in the Yellow Pages.

Charitable free clinics (private or volunteer). These clinics offer health care and drugs to the working poor. Because of the cost of diabetes drugs, some clinics do not offer them. Call to find out before you make the trip. If they don't offer diabetes drugs, ask where you can get them. Look up "clinics" in the Yellow Pages. If you can't find a free clinic, write for a national list of free clinics. (See Resources.)

Catholic Charities. This well-known national charity assists people in crisis in most cities. You can receive a chit to redeem for drugs at local pharmacies. Look up "Catholic Charities" in the white pages.

Churches. Your church may have emergency funds for drugs. Call the church office or ask your pastor.

Indigent drug program run by the Pharmaceutical Manufacturers' Association. Most drug manufacturers have assistance programs for indigent people needing the drugs that they manufacture. Most require that your physician call the company or sales representative to get you into the program. To find out if there is a program for your drug, call (800) PMA-INFO. Keep in mind that it will probably take a few weeks to get assistance from these programs. Most diabetes drug and insulin manufacturers have charitable programs. Your physician or diabetes nurse may be able to set something up for you with a drug company sales representative.

Your health-care professional. If you can't afford drugs, tell your doctor or nurse. They sometimes have free samples from the manufacturer on hand or know of emergency programs.

United Way. If you have no idea where to start, ask your local United Way workers for information about free medical care programs and food programs.

> **TIP:** Tell the receptionist at a pharmacy program that you have diabetes and need help immediately. Explain that without medication you could suffer serious health problems within a few days.

Going for Help

Once you find a pharmacy program, go prepared. Most must see evidence of your financial status. Be sure to take the following with you:

✔Income information for all wage earners in the house. Take paycheck stubs, check stubs from any pension or assistance program (unemployment, social security, retirement), or a monthly earnings statement from your employer.

✔ID or birth certificates for all household members.

✔Prescription (or bottle/vial showing your medication).

✔ A good attitude — and something to read. Remember that the case workers don't make the rules. If you are rejected for assistance, ask where you should go next. Usually, government programs refer unqualified applicants to charitable organizations such as Catholic Charities or United Way programs.

You may need help getting your diabetes drugs during and after floods, hurricanes, and other natural disasters. Insulin can spoil with no refrigeration at temperatures higher than the 80s. If this happens to you, go to a Red Cross assistance center for help. A few ADA affiliates do offer assistance during natural disasters. After disasters, you can sometimes get testing devices and strips donated by manufacturers through the Red Cross.

$ $ $ $ $ $ $
Educating Family and Co-Workers

Sometimes other people can spot trouble sooner than you can—if you've taught them how to do it. Teach your family members and co-workers the signs of low blood sugar. Naturally, you don't experience all of these. In fact, you may not have any symptoms, but tell them what to watch for. Then, ask them to do three things when they think your blood sugar is low:

✔Tell you that you might have low blood sugar. (Warn them that you may deny it and get angry.)

✔Ask you to check your blood sugar and to tell them the number. (Tell them what your normal sugar levels should be ahead of time.)

✔If your sugar level is low, they should have you drink something, such as milk or juice. Tell them to be sure you drink even if you get really angry at them. Low blood sugar levels can change your behavior, and you may not even be aware of what you are saying.

Avoiding low blood sugar is especially important if you do physical work or work with machines. You don't want to lose control—it could be dangerous.

Others can help you with high blood sugar episodes, too. Ask for help with detecting ketones. Ketones are a problem if your blood sugar tends to run high, you skip meals, or you don't take your medication. Family members or co-workers may smell ketones on your breath. This fruity-smelling odor can be mistaken for alcohol. *Do* tell co-workers about this. Explain that this odor is a sign of diabetes problems, *not* alcohol consumption.

Don't know how to approach co-workers? Ask for the ADA pamphlet *A Word to Employers* (see Resources.) $

Sacrificing Prevention:
Penny-Wise but Pound-Foolish

"The blood-testing sticks go first—the monitoring," says Dr. Lisa Wheaton, MD. She is a primary-care physician who has volunteered at two free clinics in Washington, DC.

After strips, people cut back on the number of insulin injections, oral drugs, or blood pressure medication. Low-income patients also give up on preventive medicine. They skip such things as checkups every few months and yearly eye doctor visits. "This actually leads to *more* emergency room visits," Wheaton says. By skipping routine checkups, low-income patients are more seriously ill when they get to the hospital. Sadly, many of their illnesses could have been prevented. They just had to *seek medical help earlier.*

Wheaton recalls one diabetes patient who does it right. He is a homeless man who has maintained his blood sugar levels around 200 mg/dl. "That's pretty good for someone out on the street," she says. The secret to her patient's success: He maintains a close connection with a doctor at a free clinic. He goes to see this doctor regularly. He goes whether he feels ill or not. He also continues his blood glucose tests, three times a week.

"I don't want people to think that just because they're broke, they can't maintain their diabetes properly," Wheaton said. "They can."

7

Federal and State Health and Food Programs

Our taxes help the U.S. Government, along with state and local governments, bring health and food assistance to millions of needy Americans.

Caution: Federal and state government assistance programs are in a period of major change. In early 1995, however, the programs helped

Elderly people   Poor people
Those with disabilities   American Indians
Mothers and their young children
Veterans

All of these groups include people with diabetes. You can benefit from government health-care and food programs, such as

Medicare
Medigap insurance (private)
Medicaid
Veterans Administration
Indian Health Service
Food assistance programs.

In this chapter, we outline the main features of each program. For details, call the agency. We provide 800 numbers where possible. You may want to take the time to write to your elected state and Congressional representatives. Tell them when a program helps you. Tell them that people with diabetes need to have diabetes education and assistance with the cost of supplies to live healthier lives.

Medicare

Medicare offers federal health insurance for people age 65 years and older and to some disabled people, including those with permanent kidney failure. Medicare pays some, but not all, hospital, doctor, and other medical bills.

Medicare Information

✔Call your local Social Security office or the Medicare Hot Line at (800) 638-6833 to see whether you qualify for special low-income programs.

✔Ask for the following free publications:
- *The Medicare Handbook*
- *Guide to Health Insurance for People with Medicare*
- *Medicare Savings for Qualified Beneficiaries*

Medicare is divided into two sections, A and B. Each offers a different set of medical benefits.

Part A Medicare. Most people age 65 years or older who have been employed, or whose spouse has been employed, qualify for part A Medicare.

✔You must be at least 65 years old, *or*

✔be on kidney dialysis, *or*

✔have a kidney transplant, *or*

✔have received disability from Social Security or the Railroad Retirement Board for 2 years or more.

Costs.

✔Deductibles: Annual deductibles (in 1994) were $696 for each "spell" of illness requiring hospitalization.

✔Co-payments are usually 20% of Medicare-approved costs for each service. (If your provider charges more than the approved amount, you are responsible for the additional charges.)

Coverage.

✔Medically necessary inpatient hospital care

✔Nursing home care

✔Home health and hospice care

Limitations.

✔Long illnesses: After a very long hospitalization, Medicare stops paying and you must assume responsibility for the cost. Sometimes these costs can be paid for by state Medicaid programs (see below).

✔Nursing homes: Medicare will not pay for nursing home care unless the home offers "skilled" nursing care. Do not check into a nursing home without checking with your local Medicare office to see if the home is Medicare approved.

Part B Medicare. You must purchase these benefits by paying health insurance premiums to Medicare.

Costs.

✔Premiums: In 1994, Part B premiums were $41 per month.

✔Deductibles: Annual deductible was $100 in 1994.

✔Co-payments: 20% of the cost of Medicare-covered services.

Coverage.

✔Doctor services

✔Outpatient hospital and health services

✔Durable medical equipment (some prostheses)

✔Therapeutic shoes

✔Drugs.

Help With Medicare Costs

If you qualify for Medicare but have trouble paying the insurance premiums, two other programs can help. You might be subsidized under Qualified Medicare Beneficiary (QMB) or Specified Low-Income Medicare Beneficiary (SLMB).

QMB eligibility. For the most needy applicants.

✔You must be at or below poverty-line income.

✔Monthly income must be less than $633 per person or $840 per couple. (In Alaska and Hawaii, the limits—and the cost of living—are higher.)

✔You must own no more than $4,000 in savings or investments per person or $6,000 per couple.

QMB costs. None

QMB coverage. QMB will cover

✔Your Medicare premiums

✔Medicare coinsurance

✔Medicare deductibles.

SLMB eligibility. 10% more than the QMB limits.

✔You must make less than $695 per month for one person or $922 per couple (in 1994). (Alaskan and Hawaiian limits are slightly higher.)

SLMB costs. You must pay for

✔All Medicare deductibles

✔All Medicare co-payments.

SLMB coverage. The state pays your monthly part B premium. You will still pay deductibles and copayments.

Medicare: Benefits for Diabetes

Supplies and equipment for blood sugar testing are covered

✔For people who have insulin-requiring type I or type II diabetes, not for those with non-insulin-requiring type II diabetes.

✔For those with a prescription for monitoring supplies. In addition, you must have a letter from your doctor explaining why monitoring is needed. Make many photocopies of this letter. You'll need to send a copy with every claim.

Diabetes education is covered only in some states. You must have

✔A prescription from your doctor, *and*

✔The education center must be Medicare approved.

Diabetic foot care is covered. Therapeutic shoes are covered if

✔You have a prescription, and

✔You also have a "certification of need" (see Chapter 8, Complications).

✔You cannot buy shoes from your prescribing doctor.

Diabetic eye disease laser treatment and cataract surgery are covered.

Medicare Limitations for Diabetes

Medicare will not pay for

✔Syringes or insulin

✔Insulin pumps (still considered by Medicare to be experimental)

✔Outpatient nutrition services (in most states)

✔Regular eye exams or eyeglasses.

$ $ $ $ $ $ $

Medigap Insurance Plans

Because Medicare does not cover all areas of health care, private companies offer Medigap (Medicare Supplement or Medsup) insurance. Nearly 75% of people on Medicare buy one of these private insurance plans to fill in the gaps that Medicare misses. Congress has defined 10 types of plans (A-J) that private insurance companies can offer for Medigap insurance.

Eligibility. Qualified for Medicare.

Cost. Varies with insurance company.

Medigap Information

✔Medicare Hot Line: (800) 638-6833. Ask for a copy of *Guide to Health Insurance for People with*

TIP: Since late 1994, insurance companies can legally sell you insurance policies that you don't need. The insurance agent does not have to tell you if Medicare already covers certain benefits. You could spend money on "cancer coverage" when Medicare already covers cancer at about the same rate. Consult an insurance counselor before you pay for Medigap insurance. Don't be pressured by a salesperson.

Medicare.

✔National Association for Area Agencies on Aging: (800) 677-1116.

✔National Insurance Consumer's Help Line: (800) 942-4242. Ask for a copy of *Consumer's Guide to Medicare Supplements.*

✔Private insurance agents. Before you buy a Medigap plan, decide what coverage (A-J) is best for you. Then shop around by telephone. Read policies carefully and make sure that they meet standards outlined in Medicare publications.

✔National Association of Health Underwriters: (202) 223-5533. Helps you to find a health insurance agent in your area.

✔Get rid of high-pressure salespeople.

✔Check every policy for exclusions of preexisting conditions, especially diabetes. Also check for exclusions of prescription drugs and medical equipment and supplies.

TIP: Beware of Medigap insurance sold through television, magazine, and newspaper ads. Do not buy one of these insurance programs without comparing it with other programs.

$ $ $ $ $ $ $

Medicaid

Medicaid provides a safety net for medically indigent people under age 65 years. The program combines state and federal money to pay the medical bills. It is administered by each state. Older people may also use it to supplement Medicare costs.

Each state has a different Medicaid system. Each has its own rules for eligibility, coverage, and reimbursement.

Costs. Copayments in some states.

Eligibility. You can probably qualify if you already

✔Receive Aid to Families With Dependent Children (AFDC)

✔Receive a state supplement, such as
  •Old Age Assistance
  •Aid to the Blind
  •Aid to the Permanently and Totally Disabled
  •Supplemental Security Income

✔Are a nursing home resident

✔Have end-stage renal disease (kidney failure).

Check with your local public assistance program regarding your state's Medicaid coverage, application, and eligibility.

Coverage. Medicaid may cover the same things as Medicare. Coverage is not the same in every state.

$ $ $ $ $ $ $

Veterans Administration

The Veterans Administration (VA) operates the biggest health-care system in the country.

Eligibility. Even VA officials admit that VA eligibility is a tangled maze of rules.

Vets with diabetes may be eligible for health-care services if they got diabetes during their active duty or if they are indigent. An acute episode requiring hospitalization might make a difference. You must pass income eligibility standards unless you are in one of three classes:

Mandatory. The VA must provide hospital care and possibly nursing-home care if you have a service-related health problem, are a former prisoner of war, were exposed to herbicides in Vietnam, were exposed to radiation during atmospheric nuclear testing and in the occupation of Hiroshima or Nagasaki, or are a veteran on a VA pension.

Discretionary. The VA may provide hospital or nursing home care if you are rated 0–20% for a service- or nonservice-connected condition or were exposed to toxic or radioactive substances and have a related condition. You must pay a $36 co-payment for each visit (1994).

Indigent. Income eligibility guidelines for mandatory and discretionary veterans: Incomes less than $19,912 if single or $23,987 if married or single with one dependent, plus $1,330 for each additional dependent. For information about the VA health care:

✔Call (800) 827-1000 to order the VA eligibility fact sheet and to get the 800 number for your regional VA.

$ $ $ $ $ $ $

Indian Health Service, Tribal Facilities

More than 1.33 million American Indians can receive health care from the Indian Health Service (IHS) of the Bureau of Indian Affairs (BIA). Many can also receive health care at tribal-run health facilities independent of IHS.

IHS and tribal health services are especially important for American Indians, because 30% or more of IHS clients are below the United States official poverty line. The IHS is making a strong effort to provide nutrition services, clinical help, and diabetes education at many locations.

Direct care. Hospitals, clinics, and more remote health stations. Most of these are located on reservations.

Contract care. For clients living in cities or off reservations. Provides funds for non-IHS health providers and services.

Eligibility. For direct care you must be a member of a recognized tribe. Rules for tribal membership—percent Indian ancestry, etc.—vary from tribe to tribe. Basically, you must present your BIA card.

For contract care, a BIA card is necessary. Many

rules must be followed to get payment for medical help off the reservation.

A BIA card may not be needed in some areas, especially California. Again, regulations vary from state to state and tribe to tribe.

IHS information. The IHS has no national 800 number for information. Contact your nearest BIA area office (look in the blue pages under the U.S. Government, Department of the Interior) to find out if you qualify and how to obtain care.

$ $ $ $ $ $ $

Food Assistance Programs

Food Stamps

This federal program gives coupons to needy people. These coupons can be used to pay for food in most grocery stores.

Costs. None.

Eligibility. If you are poor—even temporarily—you are probably eligible for food stamps. Eligibility depends on your family income and the bills you must pay.

Food stamp applications. Apply for stamps to be mailed monthly or for an emergency situation. Go to your city or county's public assistance office. Take along with you

✔ID (birth certificate, driver's license, social security card) for all members of your family

✔Your checking or savings account records

✔Proof of all earned and unearned income for the past 30 days for all family members

✔Proof of family costs (rent or mortgage receipts, utility bills, telephone bills, medical bills, and receipts for household members over 60 years of age or disabled, if they are not on Medicaid)

✔Proof of child-care or adult-care expenses.

Government Surplus Food

The federal government periodically trucks surplus foods to charity food programs for distribution. You never know what the food will be. It could be processed cheese, canned beans, canned meat, or peanut butter.

Costs. None.

Eligibility. The distributing agency decides. Take any food stamp or assistance, or proof of recent family income and expenses.

Distribution locations. Distributions are at different locations. Call your local public assistance office to find out where and when they take place. The food goes quickly, so get there on time.

Women, Infants, and Children (WIC) Programs

If you are pregnant or have young children, you may get food assistance from the WIC program. Not all localities have this program. It combines food assistance with pregnancy and well-baby health-care assistance. The WIC program emphasizes the purchase of highly nutritious foods such as milk.

Costs. None.

Eligibility. Low-income pregnant women and high-risk children up to the age of 5 years.

Information. Ask your local health department if WIC is available.

> TIP: It usually takes a few weeks before the food stamps show up in your mailbox. If you are in a food emergency, and **especially** if you tell the administrators that you have **diabetes**, you may be issued some emergency stamps.

Meals-on-Wheels

This program brings a daily hot meal to homebound or bedridden people or takes meals to a center. Transportation may be provided. There may be a waiting list in your community, so sign up now if you need the service.

Costs. Donation.

Eligibility. Varies from state to state.

Information. Call (800) 999-6262 for information on nutrition and meal services in your area Monday through Friday 9 AM to 4:30 PM EST. You can leave a recorded message after those hours or on weekends. **$**

8

Diabetes Complications and the Pocketbook

More than 13 million people in the United States have diabetes. According to the U.S. Census Bureau, about 1.6 million of these folks claim to be disabled by diabetes and its complications. Those complications make life with diabetes even more expensive.

$ $ $ $ $ $ $

Kidney Disease: Support From All Directions
End-stage renal disease (ESRD) is the term for complete kidney failure. ESRD qualifies you for Medicare, regardless of age. ESRD also makes it easier for low-income people to get Medicaid. It is possible to have kidney failure and still lead a relatively normal life. If you need it, however, you can receive Social Security Disability support as well.

Prevention Saves Dollars and Kidneys
The best ways to keep kidney disease costs down are to prevent kidney damage and slow its progression.

✔Lower high blood pressure. Drugs, such as captopril, not only control blood pressure but slow damage to kidneys, too.

✔Keep blood sugar near normal.

✔Your doctor may recommend other treatment. Never take any nonprescription medication without your doctor's O.K.

Treatment for kidney disease is improving every

day. All treatment options are covered by Medicare, Medicaid, private insurance, and other programs discussed below.

There are several treatments for kidney failure.

✔Kidney transplantation is the preferred option for people under 55 years old. The failed kidney is surgically replaced with a kidney from a donor.

✔Hemodialysis: Three times a week, patients spend 4 hours at the hospital or a center having a machine remove wastes from their blood.

✔Peritoneal dialysis: Patients can use an implanted pump or home dialysis system.

✔Continuous Ambulatory Peritoneal Dialysis (CAPD) is like an insulin pump. It can be worn during normal activities. Periodically patients must empty a fluid collection bag.

✔Continuous Circulating Peritoneal Dialysis (CCPD) is another home dialysis system. The patient hooks up to a bedside machine for overnight dialysis.

Information and Financial Assistance

Many sources offer free counseling and information on kidney failure treatments and financing. For addresses, phone numbers, and more information, see Resources.

U.S. Government.

✔Medicare: Ask the business manager at your clinic for help, and call your Medicare office and ask for free publications. (see Resources.)

✔ESRD Networks.

Private Organizations.

✔American Kidney Fund (AKF)

✔National Kidney Foundation (NKF)

ESRD: Who pays for what? Most patients with ESRD are covered by Medicare, regardless of age. They, or their spouses or parents, have made Social Security payments from their paychecks. Medicare, Part A, covers 100% of approved hospital costs. Part B pays 80% of medical expenses, including dialysis. (Part

66

B has a monthly premium that you must pay.)

Employee group health plans pay 80% of dialysis/transplant costs for the first 18 months of dialysis. During this time, the patient must apply for Medicare. After 18 months, Medicare pays up to 80% of the bill. Most private insurance will pay the remaining 20%. A Medigap policy may pay for your Medicare deductibles and co-payments.

Social workers and administrators at treatment centers will guide you through the insurance maze. They'll help you make applications for Medicare, insurance payments, and other assistance programs.

Medicare pays:

✔$126 (80%) per dialysis treatment in centers. (Patient or insurance pays $25.25.)

✔$130 (80%) per dialysis treatment in hospitals.

✔Home dialysis costs (ceilings set depending on method).

✔100% of kidney transplant acquisition, 80% of surgery.

✔For immunosuppressant drugs—mostly cyclosporine. After Jan. 1, 1995, 18 months of the drug will be paid. In 1996, 24 months will be paid; in 1997, 30 months; and in 1998, 36 months.

For people not eligible for Medicare, Medicaid will pay 100% of the costs. Medicaid may also cover prescription drugs and transportation.

Transportation. Many patients on dialysis have had amputations or use a wheelchair. They use county handicapped van services, city step-buses, or cabs. In most communities, local government provides transportation for people with handicaps. A clinic social worker will find a way to get you to the clinic if you have transportation problems. The American Kidney Fund (see above) may help with funds for transportation.

Almost everyone can get kidney treatment. Do not avoid seeking treatment because you have no money.

People at the clinic will help you find a way.

$ $ $ $ $ $ $

Foot Complications

Diabetes can harm your feet by damaging your nerves and blood vessels. Foot problems can be expensive if they don't get treated.

Prevention

Here are low-cost methods of preventing foot problems:

✔Wash and inspect feet daily. Dry between toes gently to remove any dry skin and lint.

✔If you can't see your feet, use a mirror, or ask a family member or friend to check your feet regularly.

✔Wear well-fitted shoes and cotton socks. Inspect your socks before and after wearing to check for drainage from sores you cannot feel.

✔Don't wear new shoes for longer than 2 hours at a time.

✔Don't wait for pain. The longer you have diabetes, the more chance you'll have nerve damage in your feet. You may not be able to feel sores, objects in your shoes, or badly fitting shoes.

✔Always ask your doctor to inspect your feet. Always tell your doctor about foot sores—even if you came about another problem.

✔Go to the doctor immediately if you have a sore that does not heal. Don't wait until it starts spreading. Sores can grow deep into your foot, where you can't see them.

✔Go to a foot clinic even if you think your foot is beyond hope. Even people with serious foot problems can be helped. A study of people with amputations showed that those who went to foot clinics had less serious amputations.

✔Invest in a pair of $20 shoe insoles. Insoles can turn a regular pair of shoes into a "comfort shoe." Buy insoles at athletic shoe stores, pharmacies, or grocery stores.

✔Invest in a comfort shoe or good athletic shoe. Comfort shoes can be purchased at a specialty shoe store. (Look in the Yellow Pages under "shoes-orthopedic.") At an orthopedic shoe store, a licensed pedorthist can fit you with an appropriate shoe. They will have off-the-shelf, nonprescription shoes costing between $80 and $90 (but shoes on sale can cost under $50).

You must see a professional to get prescription, custom-made shoes and orthotic devices. They are paid through insurance. **Note:** Nonprescription shoes may cost more in their shops.

$ $ $ $ $ $ $

Foot Care

✔Lightly moisturize your feet daily but do not get cream between your toes. You can use corn oil or shortening. If you wear support stockings, moisturize at night after you take them off.

✔Wear clean socks every day; during the heat of summer you may want to change your socks twice a day.

✔Do not use garters, elastics, or tight panty girdles.

✔Never walk barefoot on hot sand or pavement.

✔Check your bath water before getting into it. It should not be hot.

✔Never use hot water bottles or heating pads to warm your feet. If your feet get cold, wear a loose pair of socks to bed.

✔Trim nails straight across; do not round corners. You can call your local hospital to see if a foot clinic is available to you.

✔Never cut corns or calluses yourself.

✔Do not use adhesive tape on your feet.

✔Never use hot or cold soaks on your feet.

When you visit the doctor, always have your bare feet checked.

✔Go to the doctor if you develop a blister, puncture, or sore on your foot.

Treatments and Aids

Medicare and therapeutic shoes. In 1993, Congress allowed Medicare to pay for therapeutic shoes for people with diabetes. For Medicare reimbursement for custom-fitted shoes, you need:

✔a prescription from a physician or a podiatrist.

✔a letter from the prescribing doctor to certify that you need the shoes for diabetic disease.

You cannot buy the shoes from the same doctor who wrote the prescription.

Unfortunately, Medicare pays very little for therapeutic shoes. Only a few therapeutic shoe stores accept Medicare business. You may have to find some other way to pay for the shoes. Talk to people at a free clinic or charity group.

More and more private insurance companies are paying for therapeutic footwear, as are a number of state Medicaid programs.

Amputation and prostheses. In 1990, 54,000 people with diabetes had leg or foot amputations. To help you get moving after amputation, you may need artificial limbs—prostheses—or wheelchairs.

A below-the-knee prosthetic device can cost up to $8,000. An above-the-knee device costs up to $13,000. High-tech prostheses are made with lightweight materials and sophisticated joints. They offer good mobility. They also cost the most. Older, heavier prostheses will do for people who are not very mobile. They cost less.

Most people with diabetes who have amputations tend to be older and thus are covered by Medicare and secondary insurance. Other people can pay for prosthetics in a number of ways, including Medicaid.

✔State or local vocational rehabilitation offices

will help. Younger people facing amputations will find vocational rehabilitation agencies willing to pay for prostheses, especially if you can then return to work.

✔Local churches and fraternal organizations, such as the Moose Club, the Lions Clubs, or the Shriners, may offer money. Lions have dedicated funds and facilities for children with orthopedic problems.

✔Orthotic/prosthetic clinics work with low-income people. They may bill you in installments. Sometimes the bills for customers in extreme financial hardship are simply written off.

Wheelchairs. Wheelchairs vary in price from $450 to $2,000. Amputees may require an elevating leg rest and an amputee attachment that acts as a counterweight for the missing limb. These specialty items can raise the cost an additional $1,200–$1,500.

Medicare does not pay for wheelchairs—it "rents with an option to buy." Payments, or rent are divided over 15 months. For 13 months the patient pays roughly $55 a month (for a standard chair with no accessories). Later Medicare should refund the patient 80% of that rental. At 13 months, the patient makes payments for 2 more months directly to the vendor to purchase the chair. This is the only way Medicare will pay for the chair. However, few medical supply stores will take Medicare "assignment." This is because Medicare reimbursements are unreliable and take so much paperwork. You may have to pay for the chair yourself.

Your wheelchair prescription. Your doctor must write a prescription for a wheelchair so that Medicare, Medicaid, or your insurance will pay for it. If you plan to be very mobile, a sport wheelchair can get you back into the action. However, they cost $400 to $1,000 more. Medicare pays only for standard chairs.

Consider the use of chair cushions because all of your weight is now on the ischial spines.

Before your doctor writes the prescription for your

chair, discuss the lifestyle you plan to lead. Some doctors know very little about available models and attachments. Talk to a vocational rehabilitation worker or physical therapist about your wheelchair if you plan to go back to work. Check to see if the public library carries magazines for people with disabilities.

Buying a wheelchair.

✔Use the Yellow Pages. Check under "Hospital Equipment and Supplies."

✔Look for a vendor that advertises Medicare assignment.

When you are not eligible for medicare refunds.

✔Seek a business that does not sell equipment on commission. Commission-sales stores tend to have higher prices.

✔Get bids. Tell the stores what kind of chair you want and what accessories are needed. Ask for their prices. Buy the best deal you can find.

$ $ $ $ $ $ $

Eyes : Seeing Your Way to Help

Prevention. Go to an eye doctor at least once a year to head off problems that could lead to blindness.

Treatment Assistance. Medicare will not pay for routine eye examinations or glasses. Medicare does pay for cataract eye glasses, contact lenses, or inside-the-eye lenses for cataracts. See Resources for more information about these groups offering financial assistance for eye care.

National Eye Care Project. Call (800) 222-EYES (3937). The American Academy of Ophthalmology National Eye Care Project is for low-income U.S. citizens and legal residents. They provide a comprehensive eye exam and any follow-up treatment needed. You are eligible if

✔you are 65 years of age or older,

✔you are a U.S. citizen or legal resident,

✔you have not had an eye exam for the past 2 years, and

✔you do not have access to an ophthalmologist for some reason.

Doctors find a way to help patients who cannot pay.

Benevolent and Protective Order of Elks (BPOE). This fraternal organization has extensive eye programs for the needy.

Lions Club International. Call your local Lions chapter. This group sponsors various eye programs, depending on the local chapter. Your local club may support

✔Eye examinations and glasses for low-income people

✔A mobile screening van

✔A guide-dog program

✔Assistance for blind athletes and bowlers

✔Recording services.

U.S. Veterans. If you are eligible for VA medical services, you may be eligible for assistance at a VA Blind Rehabilitation Center or clinic.

Information. For information on vision loss, services, and products, see Resources for the National Eye Institute, American Foundation for the Blind (AFB), and Resources for Rehabilitaion.

$ $ $ $ $ $ $

Impotence

Sexual problems (impotence in men, loss of sensation in women) are common among people with long-term type II and type I diabetes. Good blood sugar control helps prevent or slow down development of these problems. Talk with a gynecologist or a urologist.

Impotence is not inevitable in old age. Some men and women are too embarrassed to talk to a doctor. Some doctors have a "just-live-with-it" attitude about loss of sexual function. If yours does this, find another doctor.

Diabetes can cause impotence or loss of sensation in two ways: nerve damage and hardening of the arteries. A woman with these conditions can lose feeling in sensitive tissue. In a man's case, the penis does not get enough blood to create or maintain a full erection. Diabetes can also damage tissues within the penis. High blood pressure and cigarette smoking cause additional damage.

Pumps. Pumps combine a cylinder with a pump that creates a vacuum. Blood is drawn into the penis, creating an erection. A constriction ring placed at the base of the penis prolongs the erection. If you have a prescription, insurance and Medicare will pay all or most of the $400–600 cost (Medicare pays up to 80%.). These pumps safely control the blood pressure inside the penis, and the constriction ring is pliable.

Other treatments for impotence. 1) A surgically inserted prosthesis costs $5,000 or more. 2) Injectable drugs help men with undamaged blood vessels in the penis. However, this treatment poses the risk of hours-long erections and the development of internal scar tissue.

Some men have a low-hormone condition that causes lack of sexual desire. This condition can be treated with testosterone injections. Many doctors prescribe drug treatment before recommending the pump. Discuss your options, their success records, and monthly costs with your doctor.

TIP: Medical pump models are better made than the novelty store versions. Nonprescription devices ($20–150) may be dangerous to use. It is possible to over-engorge the penis. This is especially dangerous for men who take prescription anticoagulants or aspirin, because heavy bleeding or severe bruising may occur. Also the metal constriction rings can cause tissue damage.

$ $ $ $ $ $ $

Depression and Mental Illness: Invisible Handicaps

Depression can result from extra stress or from some biochemical factor. Patients with poor glucose control may be depressed. Two other high-risk groups are those who are newly diagnosed and those who are worried about long-term complications.

The link between diabetes and eating disorders is being seen more and more. This condition requires medical help—and sometimes hospitalization.

Sometimes, the most effective way to cope is to involve the entire family in therapy. This is because family stresses add to your psychological problems. In turn, diabetes creates stresses on everyone in the family. It helps to know when depression becomes a medical problem. Signals to watch for are

Long-lasting blues

Weepiness

Sleep disturbance (too much or too little)

Lack of motivation

Feelings of deep despair, suicidal thoughts, or actions.

When these appear, get professional help. Untreated mental illness can be very costly, especially when it interferes with school, work, family relationships, and overall health.

Paying for Mental Health Professionals

Insurance companies usually pay 50% of the doctor's fees (instead of the 80% paid for other illnesses); limit the number of times per year you can have therapy, and limit the amount of hospitalization they cover.

Medicare: Stays in specialized hospitals (such as mental hospitals) are limited to 190 days. Psychiatric care in general hospitals, however, is treated the same as other hospital care. Day treatment (partial hospitalization) may be covered if approved by Medicare—it's most likely to be approved in community mental health centers and hospital outpatient departments. Be sure to check your coverage before you are hospitalized. For outpatient mental health care, Medicare matches private insurance—only 50% is covered, after deductible. Make sure that your private mental health professional has Medicare assignment.

Municipal mental health programs. Look under your public health department listings for mental health care. Even with insurance or Medicare, low-income people should look into public mental health programs. Mental health centers have psychiatrists to handle emergencies and prescribe medications and therapists for regular "talk" therapy. The centers will also offer vocational rehabilitation specialists.

TIP: If you are feeling desperate, call a crisis hot line and ask for help (look in the Yellow Pages under "crisis intervention") or call the local directory assistance operator.

Public mental health clinics usually charge on a sliding scale. If you are insured, they'll bill the insurance company. If not, you pay according to your income. Take your household income and expense records with you for your first appointment, unless it's an emergency. If you have very low income, you may receive mental health services free.

Soul solutions. Some mental health researchers have found that religion helps with depression and stress management. If you've never adopted any spiritual practice, you might consider exploring different religions. You can't beat the price.

Many clergy members are also skilled counselors. Every hospital has staff clergy from whom you can request a visit.

A little help from your friends. The best form of mental health aid can come from friends. Choose a friend who listens well—one who might even be a little tough friend who listens well—one who might even be a little tough with you. Don't pick someone living with you—they may be too close to the situation. If you can't find a friend, or are too shy to ask, talk to someone at church or to a personnel specialist at work. Many companies have mental health counseling available for employees.

AA or NA. Alcohol and drug use make it much harder to follow your diabetes treatment plan.

Alcoholics or Narcotics Anonymous meetings are free. In most cities and towns, you can find a meeting several times a day. Look in the white pages under AA, "Alcoholics Anonymous" or "Narcotics Anonymous," or in the Yellow Pages under "alcohol treatment centers." Or call the local hospital detox center or psychiatric unit. They'll have a list of nearby meetings. Or, just ask the directory assistance operator for the nearest "AA" number. Another place to check is your local mental health center. $

Hello!

Dial 411 to get the local directory assistance operator. Operators can help you find local crisis hot lines, whether it's for a family crisis, a suicide prevention, or rape crisis. The state directory assistance operator can be reached at 1-area code-555-1212.

If your local area has few crisis lines, call the toll-free information operator (800) 555-1212. Nearly every national health association has an 800 number for help or information.

9

Resources

$ $ $ $ $ $ $

General

American Diabetes Association: (800) 232-3472—1660 Duke Street, Alexandria, VA 22314.
Supports diabetes research, education, and public awareness. Annual membership ($24) brings you the monthly consumer magazine, *Diabetes Forecast.* 800 local chapters. Free educational publications to inquirers. Free catalogue of books.
American Association of Diabetes Educators: (800) 832-6874—444 N. Michigan Avenue, Suite 1240, Chicago, IL 60611. They can help you find a diabetes educator in your area.
The American Dietetic Association: (800) 366-1655—Consumer Nutrition Hot Line to locate a dietitian, talk to a dietitian, listen to recorded educational messages, or request free publications.

$ $ $ $ $ $ $

Insulin

Eli Lilly and Company: (800) 545-5979; Medical Hot Line Customer Service—Lilly Corporate Center, Indianapolis, IN 46285. Indigent Patient Program. (800) 545-6962. Have your doctor call this number for forms. You provide income information, and on approval, a 3-month insulin supply is sent to your doctor. It may be renewed.
Novo Nordisk Pharmaceutical: (800) 727-6500;

Professional Services Hot Line—100 Overlook Center, Suite 200, Princeton, NJ 08540-7810.

Indigent Patient Program: Patients can call for an application form to take to a doctor for a one-time-only, 3-month insulin supply.

Novo Nordisk has a Keeping Well With Diabetes program. Call (800) 243-3378 to join. You will receive three rebate coupons to pay for Novo insulin, a Diabetes Information Pack, and a quarterly newsletter about diabetes self-management.

$ $ $ $ $ $ $

Other Drugs

Pharmaceutical Manufacturers Association: (202) 835-3400—1100 15th Street, NW, Washington, DC 20005. Order the *Directory of Prescription Drug Patient Assistance Programs*, listing companies that donate drugs to needy patients, usually on the request of their physicians.

American Association of Retired Persons: (800) 456-2277. Call for information regarding their mail-order pharmacy program. Uninsured people and nonmembers may use the service.

Planned Parenthood: (800) 782-2859 or, look in the white pages of your phone book. They provide assistance with birth control medications.

$ $ $ $ $ $ $

Mail-Order Pharmacy and Supply Houses

Penny Saver Medical Supply: (800) 748-1909.

Preferred Rx: (800) 843-7038. (no Medicare or Medicaid).

Jocelyn Bischoff's Diabetic Depot of America Inc.: (800) 537-0404.

Hospital Center Pharmacy: (800) 824-2401.

Diabetic Care Center: (800) 633-7167.

Diabetic Promotions: (800) 433-1477.
National Diabetic Pharmacies: (800) 467-8546.
Edwards Healthcare Services: (800) 793-1995.
Thriftee Group Home Diabetes Care: (800) 258-9559.
American Medical Supplies: (800) 434-3536.
Liberty Medical Supply: (800) 762-8026.
Suncoast Pharmacy and Surgical Supplies: (800) 799-1991.

$ $ $ $ $ $ $

Monitor and Strip Manufacturers
Boehringer Mannheim Corporation: (800) 858-8072.
Cascade Medical: (800) 525-6718.
Chronimed/Supreme Medical: (800) 444-5951.
Home Diagnostics: (800) 342-7226.
LifeScan: (800) 227-8862.
MediSense, Inc.: (800) 527-3339.
Miles, Inc. (Bayer): (800) 348-8100.
Polymer Technology: (800) 877-4449.
Can-Am Care Corporation: (800) 461-7448.

$ $ $ $ $ $ $

Syringe Manufacturers
Becton Dickson (BD): (800) 866-0086.
Can-Am Care Corporation: (800) 461-7448—Cimetra
Industrial Park, Box 98, Chazy, NY 12921-0098.

$ $ $ $ $ $ $

Diabetes Publications
American Diabetes Association: (800) 232-3472—
1660 Duke Street, Alexandria, VA 33214. Or local
affiliate (in white pages). Monthly membership magazine: *Diabetes Forecast* ($24/yr). Offers free pam-
phlets, some in Spanish. Many books for sale, such as:
101 Tips to Improving Your Blood Sugar
The Fitness Book For People with Diabetes
The Take Charge Guide To Type I Diabetes

Type II Diabetes: Your Healthy Living Guide
Month of Meals 1, 2, 3, 4, and 5
The Healthy HomeStyle Cookbook
Great Starts and Fine Finishes
Savory Soups and Salads
Easy and Elegant Entrees
Quick and Hearty Main Dishes
Simple and Tasty Side Dishes.
Call the 800 number for a catalogue.

Keeping Well With Diabetes: (800) 243-3378. Novo Nordisk free diabetes newsletter, and Novolin insulin rebate coupons.

Living Well With Diabetes: Diabetes Center, Inc., (DCI Publishing), P.O. Box 739, Wayzata, MN 55391. Quarterly magazine and catalogue for discount supplies.

National Diabetes Information Clearinghouse: 301-654-3327—1 Diabetes Way, Bethesda, MD 20895.

$ $ $ $ $ $ $

Exercise Videos
Armchair Fitness Videos:(800) 453-6280—8510 Cedar Street, Silver Spring, MD 20910

$ $ $ $ $ $ $

Health Insurance
State insurance commissioner's office: blue pages of phone book. Answers for your questions about insurance companies in your state. Has a complaint department.
National Insurance Consumer Help Line: (800) 942-4242. Ask for *Guide to Medicare Supplement Insurance* (Medigap insurance).
National Association for Area Agencies on Aging:

(800) 677-1116. Free Medigap counseling for seniors.
National Association of Health Underwriters: (202) 223-5533. Helps you to find a health insurance agent in your area. You should talk to several salespeople, including an independent insurance agent who is not working for one particular company.
Health insurance agents: Yellow Pages

$ $ $ $ $ $ $

Health Care (Government Programs)
Social Security: (800) 772-1213. To find your nearest Social Security office. Make applications for Medicare and other programs by telephone through this number.
Medicare: Order free booklets from Consumer Information Center, Department 59, Pueblo, CO, 81009.

The Medicare Handbook (includes information about Medicare A and B programs and Medigap insurance).

Guide To Health Insurance for People with Medicare.

Medicare Coverage of Kidney Dialysis and Kidney Transplant Services.

Medicare Savings for Qualified Beneficiaries
Medicaid: Look in the blue pages under "public assistance," or "health department."
Medigap: See "Health Insurance."
Veterans Administration: Look under "United States Government," in the blue pages of the phone book.
Indian Health Service: Look under "United States Government, Department of the Interior" in the blue pages of the phone book.
Women, Infants and Children (WIC) Programs: Call your local health department in the blue pages.
Meals on Wheels Foundation: (800) 999-6262. For information on nutrition and meal delivery services, call from 9 AM to 4:30 PM, EST. You can leave a

recorded message after those hours or on weekends.

$ $ $ $ $ $ $

Health Care

Catholic Charities USA: (800) CARE-002. Makes emergency grants for medications, health care, and sometimes food. Look in your local telephone book for nearest office.

Free Clinic Foundation: (703) 344-8242—National Directory of Free Clinics, Free Clinic Foundation of America, Roanoke, VA 24007. To find a nearby free clinic. (Or look under "Clinics" or "Social Service Providers" in the yellow pages.)

Healthcare for the Homeless: (202) 628-5660. To find the nearest federally funded clinic serving homeless people. (Or look under "Clinics" or "Social Service Providers" in the yellow pages.)

$ $ $ $ $ $ $

Kidney Complications

U.S. Government: Order free booklet, *Medicare Coverage of Kidney Dialysis and Kidney Transplant Services*, about payment for kidney failure treatment from: Consumer Information Center, Department 59, Pueblo, CO 81009.

ESRD Networks: (804) 794-3757—MidAtlantic Renal Coalition, 1527 Hugenot Road, Midlothian, VA 23113 This government network of 18 regional organizations provides valuable information about ESRD treatment options, dialysis, and transplant centers in your community. They provide statistics that can help you choose a kidney transplant center. Call the number above for a listing of all centers, or call the American Kidney Fund Help Line (below) for your nearest center.

American Kidney Fund Help Line: (800) 638-8299—ADF, 6110 Executive Boulevard, Ste. 1010, Rockville, MD 28052. Telephone advice, free publications, referrals. Eligible patients can receive aid, after referral from treatment centers. Aid programs offer financial assistance for drugs, travel, donor travel, dialysis on travel, and oral iron medication. .

Ask for free publications:

AKF Patient Aid Programs

The American Kidney Fund Helps When Nobody Else Will

AKF Responds to Most Frequently Asked Questions.

Diabetes and The Kidneys

Kidney Disease: A Guide For Patients And Their Families

National Kidney Foundation (NKF): (800) 622-9010—30 East 33rd Street, New York, NY, 10016. Free publications about kidney disease, diabetes, diet, and other health issues. NKF has 52 state and regional affiliates, similar to the American Diabetes Association. Local affiliates offer limited financial assistance for drugs and transportation. They also have local support groups. NKF supports research and emphasizes public and professional education. The quarterly newspaper, *Family Focus,* is free.

$ $ $ $ $ $ $

Eye Complications

American Academy of Ophthalmology: (415) 561-8500—P.O. Box 7424, San Francisco, CA 94109-1336. Request information on programs to support low-income people needing eye exams and treatment.

American Foundation for the Blind (AFB): (800) 232-5463—15 West 16th Street, New York, NY 10011. This organization offers a wide range of vision services: catalogues of consumer products, publications (large print and Braille), videos, and toys. The Blind Diabetic Division can send you a list of special equipment (such as a blood glucose monitor with a sound output), books, and videos.

Benevolent and Protective Order of Elks (BPOE): The Elks run hospitals specializing in eye disease. Ask your doctor to apply for assistance on your behalf, through your local chapter (in the white pages).

Lions Club International: Local chapters run a variety of programs to prevent and treat eye disease. Call your local group (in the white pages) to see what programs they have.

National Eye Institute: (301) 496-5248—NEI, Building 31, Room 6A32, Bethesda, MD 20892. Free brochures on eye diseases, including diabetic retinopathy, cataracts, and macular degeneration.

National Foundation for the Blind: (301) 659-9314—NFB, 1900 Johnson Street, Baltimore, MD 21230. Information about laws, new technology, diabetes, etc. Catalogue of specially adapted blood glucose monitors. Publications, cassettes, videos.

Resources for Rehabilitation: (617) 862-6455—33 Bedford Street, Suite. 19A, Lexington, MA 02173. Books and publications: *Living With Low Vision: A Resource Guide For People With Sight Loss, 1993* $35.00. Comprehensive. Catalogue of disability-related books.

$ $ $ $ $ $ $

Foot Complications

American Amputee Foundation: (501)-666-2523—AAF, 3609 Arapaho Trail, Little Rock, Ark 72209. Offers limited financial support on prosthetic equipment, wheelchairs. *Ability* magazine, self-help books, guides. Legal assistance, referrals, rehabilitation.

Prescription Footwear Association: (800) 381-1167. *Care of the Diabetic Foot* (800) 333-4067. Free booklet from P.W. Minor, comfort and therapeutic shoe manufacturer.

$ $ $ $ $ $ $
Mental Health
National Alliance for the Mentally Ill (NAMI): (800) 950-NAMI—200 N. Glebe Road, Ste. 1015, Arlington, VA 22203-3754. Has 1100 local affiliates. Use 800 number to find local affiliate and to order publications.

National Clearinghouse for Alcohol and Drug Information: (800) 729-6686. Information for substance abuser or family members.

Al-Anon/Alateen Family Group Headquarters: (800) 356-9996. Local groups are in the white pages. Help for family members of alcohol abusers.

Alcoholics Anonymous World Services (AA): (212) 686-1100—P.O. Box 459 Grand Central Station, New York, NY 10163. Local groups are in the white pages. For alcohol abusers who want to stop.

Narcotics Anonymous (NA): (818) 780-3951—P.O. Box 9999, Van Nuys, CA 91409. Local groups are in the white pages. For drug abusers who want to stop.

$ $ $ $ $ $ $

Impotence
Free information available from:

POS-T-VAC: P.O. Box 1436, Dodge City, KS 67801. (800) 279-7434

ENCORE: 2300 Plantside Drive, Louisville, KY 40299-1928.

VETCO, INC: (800) 827-8382—3700 5th Ave. South, Birmingham, AL 35222.

Impotence Institute of American (IIA): 800-669-1603—8201 Corporate Drive, Suite 320, Landover, MD 20785.

$ $ $ $ $ $ $

Legal Services
Employment discrimination: Call local affiliate of American Diabetes Association in the white pages. $